This book could not have been written without the aid and agreement of two important counterparts and colleagues, Paul DiSilvestro and Michael Krychman. Both have inspired and enlightened me in the care of women with cancer, and I am tremendously grateful for their friendship and continued collaborations. I would also like to thank Chris, Kathy, and Jessica at Jones and Bartlett for the opportunity to author this book, their patience with me, and their guidance. Finally, I want to thank my partner Henry for his support and encouragement.

This book is dedicated to the women in my life: my mother, Millionita; mother-in-law, Marilyn; my four sisters, Michelle, Maerica, Precy, and Marie; my niece Stella; and most of all, to my daughter Isabelle. It is also dedicated to my aunt, Norma Dongon, who is a wife, mother, and cancer survivor. I hope to one day live in a world where cervical disease and cancer will no longer be a threat to them and to us all. Finally, a special note to all of the women who have given me the tremendous honor of being their cancer-care provider and for allowing me to participate in their care. I am a better physician because of it and, more importantly, a better person.

Don S. Dizon, MD, FACP

To my two coauthors, Paul DiSilvestro and Don Dizon:

I am grateful that you included me on this project. You have encouraged me in my career and shown me that the care of women with cancer is a lifelong commitment and learning process. Don, you have been a mentor and friend; I am thankful for your friendship and look forward to our continued collaborations. To the Jones and Bartlett team, I thank you for believing in this book. To the women who read this book and for all those who will undoubtedly benefit, let us all look forward to the day when cervical disease will be a disease we only come across with historical interest in the pages of medical textbooks.

A special thank you goes to my parents Muriel and Paul Krychman, my brother Steven, my sister-in-law Nancy, nephew Gregory, and niece Hailey for their support and encouragement. To my extended family, the Franconis, thanks for the words of support. To Lutz Hillbrich, Susan Kellogg Spadt, and Nancy Cohen, you have been extra special friends and I am thankful to have you all in my life.

This book is dedicated to the most important people in my life, John and our beautiful children Julianna Corrine and Russell Matthew; you all have blessed me with the joys of family, unconditional love, and given me the strength to succeed. You all are my heart's inspiration.

Michael Krychman, MD

Cervical cancer remains a leading cause of cancer-related death for women around the world, especially in developing countries. Despite the significant reduction in cervical cancer-related deaths in the United States since the advent of the Papanicolaou smear, there is still much progress to be made. Awareness of this disease and the benefits of screening are critically important. Looking toward the future of cervical cancer care, we hope that prevention will reduce cervical cancer-related death not only in the United States, but hopefully worldwide.

It is our hope that the answers provided to the questions raised in this book will help to raise awareness not only for those diagnosed with cervical cancer but for the families and friends supporting their loved ones during their treatment.

I would like to dedicate this book to the many courageous patients with cervical cancer I have treated over the years. For most, a cure has been achieved. For those who have lost their battle, the courage they displayed and their compassion for those around them in a time of personal crisis are inspiring. It is for the memory of these women that we continue to fight against this and other cancers.

Paul DiSilvestro, MD, FACOG

CONTENTS

Of all the female gynecologic tract tumors, it is the medical profession's approach to cervical cancer that has seen the most significant gains in medical treatment. Screening has made it a rare invasive cancer in women and highly curable, given its early detection with the Pap test. For those with invasive cancers, treatment using a combination of chemotherapy and radiation is highly effective, and most women can expect treatment for cure. Now there is even hope that vaccination against the human papillomavirus will dramatically reduce the chances of finding precancerous changes in the cervix so that women will not have to face the hardships associated with repeat biopsies, diagnoses of worrisome changes, and more invasive procedures and would ultimately be spared from the diagnosis of invasive cervical cancer.

The diagnosis of cervical cancer can be a confusing one, as can be the attempts to explain the changes of the cervix in a way that most women (and even some clinicians) can understand. The treatments are numerous and the options can lead to much confusion. *100 Questions & Answers About Cervical Cancer* provides a much-needed primer for patients and their families and aims to address the questions most relevant to a woman following a diagnosis of preinvasive changes or invasive cervical cancer.

The approach to this topic has taken the collaboration of three providers who together have sought to explain the diagnosis from different points of view: medical, surgical, and psychosocial. It is our hope that this multidisciplinary approach to the diagnosis and treatment of cervical cancer will enforce the idea that a woman facing cancer is still a woman, not just a cancer diagnosis. Implied in this is our explicit statement that a woman with cervical cancer should have the disease placed in context of the woman, as a survivor. Therefore, the diagnosis and therapy share the same emphasis as that of female survivorship. To stress this point, we are honored that Darlene Leddy has provided a much-needed personal perspective of this disease. Her input lends a personal touch on this disease and shows that despite challenging circumstances, one cannot only persevere and survive, but also prosper.

We hope that this manual provides a useful starting guide for any woman diagnosed with cervical changes and those with cervical cancer. Please know that we have tried to make this book as comprehensive as possible. All sections will not be relevant to every reader, but we hope to shed some light on the disease and its treatment for women in every stage of the disease. Education is power, and we seek to empower the woman living with or at risk for cervical cancer.

PART ONE

The Basics

Where is the cervix?
What does it do?

What is cancer?

Is cancer contagious?

More . . .

1. Where is the cervix? What does it do?

This will serve as a good starting point to discuss cervical cancer and precancer. The ovaries, fallopian tubes, and uterus are what make up a woman's internal reproductive organs (**Figure 1**) and lie deep in the pelvis where they are connected to one another. The **cervix** is a part

Cervix

From the Latin for neck, it is the lowermost part of the uterus that protrudes into the vagina.

THE BASICS

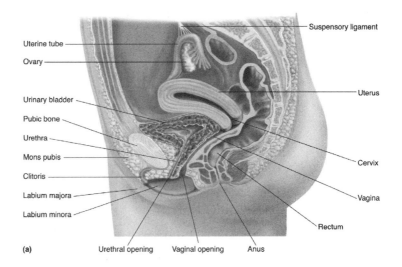

(a)

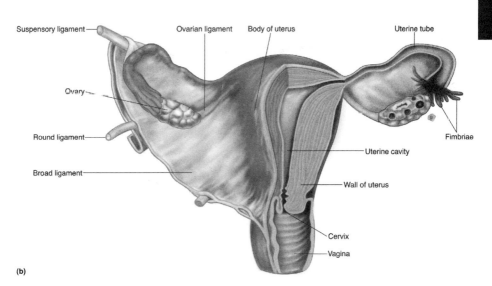

(b)

Figure 1 The female reproductive organs

Vagina

That part of the female genital tract that connects the uterus to the external vulva.

External os

The opening that connects the uterus and cervix to the vagina.

Internal os

The internal narrowing of the uterine cavity that serves as a passageway from the external os into the uterus.

The cervix functions as a passageway into and out of the uterus.

Endocervical canal

See cervical canal.

Uterus

The female reproductive organ in which pregnancy occurs.

Menopause

The permanent end of a woman's menstrual cycle.

Cervical canal

Also known as the endocervical canal, it is the tunnel that connects the uterus to the vagina.

of the uterus that extends into the vaginal vault. As such, it can be visualized when a woman has a pelvic examination. The opening to the cervix is visible in the **vagina** and is called the **external os**. There is a passageway connecting the external os to the **internal os**, the upper limit of the cervix, called the **endocervical canal** (**Figure 2**). The areas of the external os and endocervical canal are tested when a woman undergoes a Pap test.

The cervix functions as a passageway into and out of the **uterus**. For women who are not in **menopause**, it allows blood to flow out of the uterus and into the vagina where it is discarded. When a woman is having sex with a man, the cervix allows the passage of sperm into the uterus, where eggs are fertilized and pregnancy can occur. During labor, the **cervical canal**, which is usually very narrow, widens to allow the birth of a baby to take place.

The cervix also produces mucus, which serves to protect infections from reaching the upper female organs (uterus,

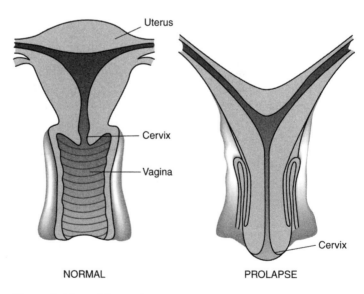

Figure 2 View of the cervix

4

fallopian tubes, and ovaries) and into the pelvic cavity. Production of this mucus is guided by female hormones during the menstrual cycle. For example, when **estrogen** is produced, this mucus is thinned, which allows sperm to enter the uterus to fertilize the egg for possible pregnancy.

Darlene's comment:

The cervix is located between the top of the vagina and at the base of the uterus. It acts as a channel to help eliminate blood from the uterus when we menstruate. It is also part of the birthing canal and dilates during labor.

2. What is cancer?

Before talking about cervical cancer or precancer, it is important to understand what cancer is—and what it is not.

What Cancer Is

Cancer results when a cell starts to grow out of control. Normally, cells follow the same cycle of growth, cell division, and eventual death. When we were still developing, first as babies inside our mothers and continuing on while we were infants and children, our cells rapidly grew and divided. The end result was **differentiation**— it's what enabled a red blood cell to carry oxygen, an intestinal cell to absorb food, and an ovary cell to produce hormones to make eggs. If cells are injured or get too old, they undergo a process called **apoptosis**, or programmed cell death. This is what keeps us healthy and all our organs operating normally.

If a cell undergoes changes in its building blocks, called **DNA**, it can escape this tightly regulated life cycle.

Estrogen
A steroid hormone produced mainly in the ovaries; it is the primary female sex hormone.

Cancer results when a cell starts to grow out of control.

Cancer
A disease characterized by uncontrolled cell growth that ultimately causes destruction of normal healthy tissue.

Differentiation
The biologic process by which a cell becomes a specific type.

Apoptosis
The process of programmed cell death.

DNA
Deoxyribonucleic acid, the building blocks of cells.

THE BASICS

5

Mutations

Cellular changes that can predispose to developing cancer.

Tumor

A cancerous mass.

Metastatic

Cancer that has spread beyond the place where it started.

These DNA changes, also called **mutations**, can allow cells to keep growing and dividing. They no longer respond to your body's signals to stop dividing, and this process of unchecked cell division results in a mass of such cells, called a **tumor**. If a tumor cell breaks free from its origin (in this case, the ovarian cell within the ovary), it can travel through the bloodstream and land in another area of one's body far away (in the lung, for example) and start growing there; it is by definition **metastatic**. These two features—unchecked cell growth and the ability to metastasize—define cancer.

What Cancer Isn't

It's important to state at this point that cancer is *not* something that can be passed from one person to another, like a virus or bacteria; cancer is not an infectious disease. You can't get cancer from another person, nor can you give it to someone else by simply coming into contact with that person, even close contact. A lot of factors contribute to the development of cancer, and in later sections we will review these risk factors and cofactors that are associated with getting cervical cancer. Most important, cancer is *not* an automatic death sentence. That's a reaction many people have because, for decades, the medical profession lacked effective treatments for most kinds of cancers, and significant fear and stigma were attached to cancer. Thankfully, medicine has come a long way and, although cancer is still a fearsome thing, many people survive it, and some are completely cured. Innovations in treatment and new drugs are developed continually, so that even the most dangerous forms of cancer are becoming increasingly curable as new information about how cancer works is uncovered.

How Cancer Spreads

Cancer can spread in three ways: by extending into surrounding tissue; by passing through the blood supply, a process called **hematogenous dissemination**; or by traveling in the **lymphatic system**, the "cleaning system" of the body, in a process termed **lymphatic spread**. Knowing the ways in which cancers spread is important, because such knowledge often is used to decide what type of surgery is necessary and what other types of treatment are necessary (such as the use of chemotherapy and the number of cycles needed).

3. Is cancer contagious?

No, cancer is not contagious. However, there are several factors that are associated with an increased risk of developing cervical cancer. One of the most important is infection with the **human papillomavirus (HPV)**, which is transmitted by sexual contact. So although cervical cancer itself cannot be spread, viral infection associated with cervical cancer can be. Later on in this book, other factors including viral infection will be discussed.

4. How do you screen for cervical cancer?

Fortunately, cervical disease can be detected even before it becomes cancer by the **Papanicolaou (Pap) test**. Introduced in 1943, the Pap test is routinely used in the United States and has resulted in a dramatic reduction in the numbers of women dying of cervical cancer by almost 75 percent.

A Pap test is performed by inserting a **speculum** into the vagina, which enables your doctor to see the cervix deep within the vaginal vault. Using a tiny spatula or

Hematogenous dissemination
The process by which cancer spreads through the bloodstream to other parts of the body.

Lymphatic system
A network of channels, nodes, and vessels that function as a transport system of lymph fluid. It functions as a major component of the immune system.

Lymphatic spread
The use of the body's filtration system by cancer cells to spread.

Human papillomavirus (HPV)
The virus associated with genital tract infections, including most cases of cervical dysplasia and cancer.

Papanicolaou (Pap) test
A cervical test that is used to screen for cervical changes or cancer.

Speculum
A medical examination tool that enables a doctor to view the cervix.

THE BASICS

7

swab, a sample of the cervix can be obtained, which is then put on a glass slide and sent to the laboratory. Typically, the Pap test will evaluate for the presence of precancerous cervical lesions, but cervical cancer can also be identified.

The American College of Obstetricians and Gynecologists recommends a first Pap test at about 3 years following your first sexual experience or by age 21, whichever comes first. Beginning at around age 30, annual Pap testing is recommended. If after the age of 33, consecutive yearly Pap tests are negative, then Pap tests can be obtained every 2 to 3 years. Recent advances in science have made testing of the Pap test with another test for high-risk HPV (see **Question 6**). If both are negative, then repeat testing using this combination every 3 years also is reasonable. For women who had a hysterectomy due to noncancerous reasons, Pap tests may be discontinued.

These guidelines do not pertain to women with other medical conditions who may be at a higher risk for cervical changes or cancer. These include women with human immunodeficiency virus (HIV), those on medicines that affect the immune system, or those who had a prior history of cervical cancer, for example.

5. How big of a problem is cervical cancer in the United States? What about internationally?

Within the United States, precancerous lesions are far more common than cervical cancer. Approximately 50 million women undergo a Pap test each year, of which 7 percent have some type of abnormality requiring the evaluation. Low-grade lesions of the cervix are diagnosed in approximately one million women, while an additional 500,000 may have higher grade lesions, which would require further evaluation.

Invasive cervical cancer is not a common cancer in women within the United States. Approximately 11,000 women are diagnosed with cancer of the cervix each year, but a little over 3500 women die of cervical cancer. Fortunately, the death rate from cervical cancer has declined in the United States by 4 percent per year.

Unfortunately, the worldwide incidence of cervical cancer is much more striking, with 83 percent of cervical cancers in the developing countries. Worldwide, 510,000 women will be diagnosed with cervical cancer, with 280,000 dying of their disease. The highest incidence rates are observed in sub-Saharan Africa, Melanesia, Latin America, the Caribbean, and within south-central and southeast Asia. The large burden of disease is likely due to the lack of cancer prevention programs within developing countries.

The death rate from cervical cancer has declined in the United States by 4 percent per year.

THE BASICS

9

PART TWO

Risk Factors and Cofactors

Are there risk factors
for cervical cancer?

How is sexual activity associated
with a risk for cervical cancer?

Can use of birth control pills increase
my risk of cervical cancer?

More . . .

6. Are there risk factors for cervical cancer?

Many factors are associated with developing cervical cancer. Among the most important is infection with high-risk human papillomavirus (HPV), now understood to have a central role in the development of cervical cancer. In addition to HPV infection, however, researchers have identified other cofactors that appear to be important to the development of cervical cancer. Among these are indicators of sexual activity, including the number of sexual partners, age at first intercourse, number of pregnancies, and a history of sexually transmitted diseases.

Other factors identified include cigarette smoking, being exposed to diethylstilbestrol while your mother was pregnant with you, and infection with human immunodeficiency virus (HIV). Finally, an increased risk of cervical cancer appears to be seen in older women, especially of non-Caucasian descent, those of lower socioeconomic status, and in women with less than a high school education.

7. How is sexual activity associated with a risk for cervical cancer?

Studies show that infection with HPV follows the parameters of sexual activity just mentioned. Although nonsexual transmission has been suggested, it has been shown that female virgins are rarely HPV infected, which argues against such nonsexual transmission of this virus.

8. Can use of birth control pills increase my risk of cervical cancer?

One risk factor that has been examined is that of oral contraceptive use. However, women using oral contraceptives tend not to use other barrier methods and also may have more sexual contacts. This makes an association between birth control pills and cervical cancer not entirely clear. A recent analysis of the literature concluded that there may be a two-fold increased risk for developing cervical cancer among women using oral contraceptives for greater than 10 years.

Darlene's comment:

Using birth control pills can increase your chances of cervical cancer, because if you are on the pill, then you are probably not using a condom and are probably more sexually active. I was on birth control when I was diagnosed with cervical cancer.

9. How is HIV related to cervical cancer?

Dysplasia
Abnormal changes in cells.

The association between abnormal cervical changes (or **dysplasia**) and cervical cancer associated with HIV has been well-known since the 1990s. Studies at that time showed that as many as 40 percent of HIV-infected women had cervical dysplasia identified by Pap test, compared to only 17 percent among non-HIV-infected women. In 1993, the Centers for Disease Control and Prevention designated moderate and severe cervical dysplasia as early evidence for symptomatic HIV infection. The onset of invasive cervical cancer is a condition that defines AIDS.

Still, even among HIV-positive women, the majority of cervical lesions in women are low grade. As in the general population, multiple factors appear to impact the risk of developing cervical dysplasia or cancer in HIV-positive women including coinfection with HPV (reportedly as high as 95 percent in this population), low CD4 counts, and high viral loads of HIV.

10. How is HPV associated with cervical cancer?

HPV is the single most important biologic risk factor for developing both precancerous lesions and invasive cancer of the cervix. Virtually all cervical cancers are causally related to viral infection with HPV. Estimates place the number of people within the United States infected with HPV at 20 million with approximately half of those age 15 to 25 years. By age 50, up to 80 percent of sexually active women will be infected with HPV. Regarding genital HPV infection, transmission is via vaginal or anal contact, but intercourse may not be necessary for transmission. This being said, nonpenetrative genital transmission of HPV is rare.

HPV is the single most important biologic risk factor for developing both pre-cancerous lesions and invasive cancer of the cervix.

The virus works by merging with the DNA in human cells. Among other things, this leads to the expression of two HPV proteins, E6 and E7, that can wreak havoc with the normal cell functions and lead the cells to the path of cancer development.

11. Are there different types of HPV?

Yes, there are multiple types of HPV strains, and more than 100 have been described. Of these, 14 are currently considered cancer causing, or high-risk types. The two most prevalent HPV strains that cause invasive cervical cancer in the United States are strains 16 and 18. However, all types of HPV can cause mild Pap test abnormalities.

12. Can you test for HPV?

The Pap test enables your doctor to test for changes in the cervix, which may be related to HPV. However, the Pap test will not tell you if cervical changes mean you have an HPV infection.

RISK FACTORS AND COFACTORS

15

There is a test that checks for HPV DNA, the genetic material of the virus itself. It is generally indicated as a follow-up test if a Pap test returns with an abnormal result. The HPV-DNA test can determine whether a high-risk type of HPV caused the abnormal Pap test. Women with a normal Pap test and no HPV infection have a very low risk for developing cervical cancer. However, those women with both an abnormal Pap test and a positive HPV test have a risk of or above 6 percent for developing cervical cancer. The Food and Drug Administration currently approves the HPV-DNA test as a screening test used with the Pap test in women over the age of 30. However, it does not substitute for regular Pap tests nor is it intended as a screen for women under 30.

13. Does HPV cause cervical cancer only?

Most HPV types cause no symptoms and will resolve on their own. However, high-risk HPV types are not only associated with cervical cancer but are also associated with less common cancers including those of the anus, vagina, and vulva. Some types of HPV may cause warts on the vagina or on the anus. The two most commonly associated with genital warts are HPV 6 and 11. In addition to genital cancers, cancers of the head and neck, including those of the soft palate, tonsils, and tongue, are also HPV related. Infection may be a risk factor for the development of penile cancer in men.

14. How long does it take to develop cervical cancer?

It is known that infection with high-risk HPV types can lead to both low-grade and high-grade changes within cervical cells. The evolution from infection with

HPV to development of a persistent infection to pre-cancerous transformation to outright cervical cancer has been estimated to take 20 years or longer. This relatively slow progression is at the root of the success of cervical cancer–screening programs.

RISK FACTORS AND COFACTORS

PART THREE

Screening and Early Cervical Changes

What is a Pap test?

How does a Pap test detect cervical cancer?

If a Pap test comes back abnormal, does it mean I have cancer?

More . . .

15. What is a Pap test?

The Pap test is a procedure done during a pelvic examination. It is performed at both gynecology and primary care physician's offices. It involves a speculum exam which allows your doctor to see the cervix. Once the cervix is seen, a spatula or a brush is used to scrape the cervix surface and the os. The scrapings then are placed on a glass slide and processed by a pathologist for further review for changes in the cells.

16. How does a Pap test detect cervical cancer?

The Pap test allows your doctor to look at the cells that line the cervix and the cervical canal. It has proven to be very effective to pick up changes in the cervix that might become cancer if left on their own. Ideally then, the Pap test allows doctors to detect cervical changes *before* they can become cervical cancer. It has proven to be one of the most effective cancer screening tests and is responsible for the decline in invasive cervical cancer in the United States.

Cellular changes are classified using the Bethesda Pap Test Classification System (**Table 1**). General categories in the Bethesda system are "negative for intraepithelial lesion or malignancy," "epithelial cell abnormality," or "other." If an **epithelial cell abnormality** is found, it is described as a **squamous** cell or a **glandular** cell. Squamous epithelial findings are further characterized into atypical squamous cells of undetermined significance or cannot exclude high-grade squamous intreaepithelial lesion; low-grade squamous intraepithelial lesion; high-grade squamous intraepithelial lesion; or squamous cell carcinoma. Glandular epithelial findings include

The Pap test allows doctors to detect cervical changes before they can become cervical cancer.

Epithelial cell abnormality

A result that may be reported on a Pap test that signifies a change is present in cells that might require further evaluation by the doctor.

Squamous

A type of cell that lines the skin and external body surfaces.

Glandular

Of or pertaining to a gland.

Table 1   The Bethesda Pap Test Classification System

The 2001 Bethesda System (Abridged)

SPECIMEN ADEQUACY

Satisfactory for evaluation (*note presence/absence of endocervical/transformation zone component*)
Unsatisfactory for evaluation...(*specify reason*)
    Specimen rejected/not processed (*specify reason*)
    Specimen processed and examined, but unsatisfactory for evaluation
        of epithelial abnormality because of (*specify reason*)

GENERAL CATEGORIZATION (Optional)

Negative for intraepithelial lesion or malignancy
Epithelial cell abnormality
Other

INTERPRETATION/RESULT

Negative for Intraepithelial Lesion or Malignancy
Organisms
    Trichomonas vaginalis
    Fungal organisms morphologically consistent with *Candida* species
    Shift in flora suggestive of bacterial vaginosis
    Bacteria morphologically consistent with *Actinomyces* species
    Cellular changes consistent with herpes simplex virus
Other nonneoplastic findings (*optional to report; list not comprehensive*)
    Reactive cellular changes associated with inflammation
        (*includes typical repair*) radiation intrauterine contraceptive device
    Glandular cells status posthysterectomy
    Atrophy

Epithelial Cell Abnormalities
Squamous cell
    Atypical squamous cells (ASC) of undetermined significance
        (ASC-US) cannot exclude HSIL (ASC-H)
    Low-grade squamous intraepithelial lesion (LSIL)
        encompassing: human papilloma virus/mild dysplasia/cervical
        intraepithelial neoplasia (CIN) 1
    High-grade squamous intraepithelial lesion (HSIL)
        encompassing: moderate and severe dysplasia, carcinoma in situ;
        CIN 2 and CIN 3
Squamous cell carcinoma
Glandular cell
    Atypical glandular cells (AGC) (*specify endocervical, endometrial, or not otherwise specified*)
    Atypical glandular cells, favor neoplastic (*specify endocervical or not otherwise specified*)
    Endocervical adenocarcinoma in situ (AIS)
    Adenocarcinoma
Other (*List not comprehensive*)
    Endometrial cells in a woman 40 years of age

AUTOMATED REVIEW AND ANCILLARY TESTING
(Include as appropriate)

Source: Adapted from Solomon D, Davey D, Kurman R, Moriarty A, O'Connor D, et al. The 2001 Bethesda System: Terminology for Reporting Results of Cervical Cytology. *JAMA*. 2002; 287(16):2114–2119.

atypical glandular cells, endocervical adenocarcinoma in situ, or adenocarcinoma.

17. If a Pap test comes back abnormal, does it mean I have cancer?

No, an abnormal Pap test does not automatically mean you have invasive cervical cancer. However, depending on the degree of abnormality, you may be recommended to undergo further testing, such as HPV-DNA testing. If a high-risk HPV was found by this DNA test, further work-up could be recommended. If not, repeat Pap testing would be performed in 12 months. If high-grade lesions were found, a **colposcopy** and/or a biopsy would be recommended.

An abnormal Pap test does not automatically mean you have invasive cervical cancer.

18. What is ASCUS? What about AGUS? Are they the same thing?

ASCUS stands for atypical squamous cells of unknown significance and AGUS for atypical glandular cells of unknown significance. ASCUS is generally considered a noncancerous finding. Atypical in this context means that the pathologist has found evidence of "irritation" but not enough to make a diagnosis of dysplasia. Approximately 70 percent of ASCUS lesions will revert to normal without anything further required. Although 7 percent may progress to higher grade over the next 2 years, the risk of progression to invasive cancer is very, very low. If ASCUS was found, repeat Pap tests may be recommended at 4 or 6 months.

As noted, AGUS refers to glandular atypical cells. These are often more concerning, and between 20 percent and

Colposcopy

A diagnostic procedure performed by gynecologists to look at the cervix more closely. It is performed with a colposcope, which is a large electric microscope that helps the doctor see the cervix more closely.

SCREENING AND EARLY CERVICAL CHANGES

Cervical intraepithelial neoplasia (CIN)

Abnormal cell growth within the cervix. It can range from low-risk changes (CIN-1) to more abnormal changes (CIN-2 and CIN-3). These are also referred to as squamous intraepithelial lesions. Although not cancer, these changes can progress into cancer.

Excision

Removal of an area of concern (whether it be an area of tumor growth or of abnormal growth) usually done with surgery.

Ablation

Removing tissue by surgery or any other means.

Hysterectomy

The surgical removal of the uterus.

50 percent of women with this diagnosis may have a more severe lesion present, which if untreated could progress into cancer. Therefore, further work-up may be indicated after it is found; usually this means a colposcopy, which would allow your doctor to sample the endocervical canal. Further evaluation with a cone biopsy may be indicated.

19. What is cervical intraepithelial neoplasia?

Cervical intraepithelial neoplasia (CIN) is another term for cervical dysplasia. Basically this means that the normally uniform layers of cells seen within the cervix are not present. CIN is classified based on the degree of dysplasia into CIN-I (low grade) or CIN-II or CIN-III (high grade). CIN-III is also referred to as *carcinoma in-situ*. These findings are based on biopsies. Of these, CIN-III correlates strongly with infection with high-risk HPV. CIN is not the same as invasive cervical cancer, but does represent preinvasive cervical carcinoma. High-grade CIN (CIN-II and CIN-III), however, requires **excision** of the affected area which can be done either through multiple techniques, including **ablation** or **hysterectomy**. The various approaches of surgical therapy for preinvasive lesions will be discussed elsewhere in the text.

PART FOUR

Treatment of Abnormal Pap Tests

How are abnormal cervical
findings treated?

What is a colposcopy?

What is a cone biopsy?
When do you have to do this?

More . . .

20. How are abnormal cervical findings treated?

Abnormal cervical findings are treated based on multiple factors. The first is the age of the patient. It has been shown that as women get older, the rates of persistence of human papillomavirus (HPV) and precancerous change (dysplasia) of the cervix increase. In older women, especially those who have completed childbearing, treatment is more likely to include an active intervention such as surgery. The second is the patient's desire for fertility. A decision to perform a procedure on the cervix of a woman who wishes to have babies in the future must take into account the impact a procedure may have on the cervix. On rare occasions, a surgery may make it more difficult for a woman to carry a pregnancy for its full length. The third factor is the severity of the abnormal cervical finding. In the lowest grades of precancerous change (dysplasia), the abnormality has a much higher likelihood of going away on its own, especially in women who are not smokers and have no significant problems with their body's immune system. As the severity of the abnormal cervical finding increases, the likelihood of the abnormality going away on its own decreases, so therefore watchful waiting is not as commonly used.

Taking these into account, a young woman who is a nonsmoker and otherwise healthy with a mild abnormality on the cervix can be observed with the knowledge that the majority of these abnormalities will go away on their own. Conversely, an older woman with a more severe abnormality on the cervix would be recommended to have surgical intervention such as a loop electrosurgical excision procedure (LEEP) or a cone biopsy (see **Question 22**).

TREATMENT OF ABNORMAL PAP TESTS

21. What is a colposcopy?

A colposcopy exam is a method of more closely evaluating the cervix of a woman with an abnormal Pap test. A colposcopy in combination with a biopsy is considered the best way to see if there is a precancerous or cancerous change of the cervix. Basically, colposcopy is a magnified view of the cervix utilizing a machine called a colposcope, which is a high-power magnifying glass. The exam is performed in a fashion quite similar to obtaining a Pap test with the patient lying on her back with feet in stirrups and an instrument called a speculum inserted into the vagina. The cervix is gently wiped clean with a large Q-tip, and then either a diluted acetic acid solution (vinegar) or a substance called Lugol's solution (iodine) is applied to the cervix. The healthcare provider then looks through the colposcope at the cervix.

Transformation zone

The area in the cervix marked by the transition between the outside of the cervix (lined by squamous cells) and the cervical canal (lined by columnar cells). It is also known as the squamo-columnar junction.

During the exam, the healthcare provider is looking for two important findings on the cervix. First, the provider needs to see the entire **transformation zone** of the cervix. The transformation zone (much like a border between two different surfaces) is the place on the cervix where the glandular cells that line the inside of the cervix meet the smooth skin cells that line the outside of the cervix. It is at that border that cells undergo change (transform) from one type of cell to the other. During their transformation, cells are open to damage by outside influences such as HPV. Because of this, the transformation zone is the area of the cervix that is most commonly the site of precancerous or cancerous change. By seeing the entire transformation zone, the provider can be certain that the examination is adequate to make a judgment whether there are any abnormal areas.

Identifying an abnormal lesion is aided by using acetic acid (white change) or Lugol's solution, which marks changes with color; with acetic acid, the changes appear white; if Lugol's is used, there is a lack of brown staining. If a lesion is identified, a biopsy of the cervix at that site is performed. Oftentimes after the biopsy, the provider will apply a substance, such as Monsel's solution, ferric subsulfate, to the biopsy site to stop any bleeding. After the application of this substance, many women report a blackish discharge, which is normal and to be expected.

Colposcopy is performed in excess of one million times per year in the United States and is a well-tolerated and proven method for evaluating for precancerous change of the cervix.

Darlene's comment:

A colposcopy is performed by a gynecologist and is a procedure that magnifies the surface of the cervix. The doctor swabs the surface of the cervix with a chemical to see if there is a reaction. If there is a reaction, then the doctor takes a biopsy of the area of concern. During my colposcopy, I was told that I had cervical cancer by my doctor, just on the basis of how it looked and the reaction of my cervix to the chemical. The biopsy later proved that I indeed had cervical cancer.

Colposcopy is performed in excess of one million times per year in the United States and is a well-tolerated and proven method for evaluating for precancerous change of the cervix.

22. What is a cone biopsy? When do you have to do this?

A cone biopsy is a surgical technique used in precancerous conditions of the cervix for both diagnosis and treatment. Cone biopsies can be done different ways, as

Cold knife cone biopsy

Also known as a cone biopsy, this technique enables sampling of abnormal cervical tissue that is seen during examination by the use of a scalpel. A cone-shaped portion of the cervix is removed.

Laser

A technique in which light is the source for vaporizing and removing abnormal tissue.

Loop electrosurgical excision procedure (LEEP)

A surgical technique in which an electrically charged loop of wire is passed across the surface of the cervix, resulting in the removal of abnormal tissue.

an office procedure or requiring anesthesia and a trip to the operating room.

A cold-knife cone biopsy is performed in an operating room. The term **cold knife** refers to the fact that the tissue is excised with a scalpel. A **laser** cone biopsy usually is done in an operating room although it can be performed in the office setting. Tissue is excised using a laser beam as the method of cutting. A **loop electrosurgical excision procedure (LEEP)** cone biopsy uses electrical energy conducted through a wire loop to excise tissue.

Regardless of the technique utilized, the goal of a cone biopsy is to obtain enough tissue from both the outside and inside of the cervix to help diagnose precancerous change of the cervix. Sometimes, a woman will have an abnormal Pap test but no precancerous change is seen on the cervix. In this case, the area of concern may be further inside the cervix. Because this area is difficult to see, a cone biopsy is performed.

There are several reasons why a woman would need to have a cone biopsy. The first reason is to address any discrepancy or a mismatch on prior testing. For example, a woman may have a highly abnormal Pap test, but the colposcopy does not reveal any changes visible on the outside of the cervix. The practitioner must presume that there is a problem higher up in the cervix and, hence, proceeding with a cone biopsy is indicated. Another reason would be that invasive cancer is suspected. In that situation, a cold-knife cone biopsy is indicated because it gives the best tissue specimen to be analyzed. A third would be the presence of an area of precancerous change seen at a colposcopy that extends up into the cervical canal beyond the view of the colposcope. A cone biopsy may be needed if the doctor is not able to see the entire transformation zone at the time of colposcopy. This can sometimes occur in older patients or in those who have had prior surgery on their cervix. Yet another commonly cited reason is abnormal cells on an **endocervical curettage (ECC)**, a scraping of the inside of the cervix. If an ECC has abnormal cells, then there may be an area of precancerous change higher up in the cervix beyond the view of the colposcope.

Risks of cone biopsy include risks associated with any anesthesia, although the length of the procedure is less than other common operations. Most surgeons would consider a cone biopsy to fall into the category of a minor surgical procedure. However, on rare occasions, patients may have an infection after the surgery requiring antibiotics or can experience bleeding. The most common long-term side effect of concern for women is the impact that cone biopsy will have on their ability to become pregnant or maintain a pregnancy. A single cone biopsy has not been shown to decrease a woman's ability to become pregnant and rarely does it predispose a woman to lose a pregnancy as it proceeds. Sometimes, in women who have had more than one cone biopsy, a stitch (or **cerclage**) is placed in the cervix after they become pregnant to help strengthen the cervix for the remainder of the pregnancy. An ultrasound can help to determine if a woman will need a cerclage. Due to the need for this type of evaluation, women with a history of a cone biopsy who become pregnant should see an obstetrician early in pregnancy.

23. If a part of the cervix needs to be removed, how is this done?

Based on results from a colposcopy and a biopsy, there are times when a woman will need to have a part of the cervix removed. This is usually done by a LEEP. A

Endocervical curettage (ECC)
A sampling of the internal cervix obtained during a colposcopy. The sampling is taken by scraping the inner portion of the cervix, which cannot be seen during a pelvic exam.

The most common long-term side effect of concern for women is the impact that cone biopsy will have on their ability to become pregnant or maintain a pregnancy.

Cerclage
A stitch placed into and around the cervix of a pregnant woman to help reduce the possibility of miscarriage.

LEEP is a minor surgical procedure generally performed in a physician's office or in an outpatient surgical setting. The procedure is performed with the patient in the same position as when performing a Pap test. The physician injects the cervix with a numbing agent and sometimes will put either acetic acid (vinegar) or Lugol's solution (iodine) on the cervix to help outline the area of the cervix that needs to be excised. A gel pad for grounding is placed on the patient's leg, in preparation for the electrical energy that will be used. Using a wire loop powered with electrical cutting energy, the surgeon can remove the concerning portion of the cervix. The size of the area removed depends on how much of the cervix is of concern. The actual excision lasts only about 3 to 5 seconds, with the majority of the time of the procedure involved in setup and in making certain that the patient does not bleed after the excision is complete.

Another method of removing a portion of the cervix uses the energy of a laser. A laser converts electromagnetic energy into light energy that can vaporize tissue. A woman having a laser vaporization of the cervix requires numbing medicine into the cervix, much like a LEEP, unless done under spinal or general anesthesia. Sometimes, due to the length of the procedure and the scarcity of laser machines in physician offices, the procedure is done in an outpatient surgical setting. This type of procedure usually takes 15 to 30 minutes after setup is complete.

Cryotherapy

The treatment of abnormal tissue by freezing.

The other method of removing a portion of the cervix is the use of **cryotherapy**. Cryotherapy (freezing of the cervix) was the most common method of treating precancerous lesions of the cervix before the advent of LEEP. Cryotherapy generally is performed in a physician's office. This procedure usually does not require numbing medicine and takes either a 5-minute application or two 3-minute applications.

Of the three, only the LEEP procedure will enable the surgeon to obtain a specimen that can be analyzed. However, it requires local anesthetic. Laser takes a greater amount of anesthetic than the other two but also does not produce a specimen. It is best suited to target unusually shaped lesions in the outer part of the cervix or vagina.

24. Are there any risks if you have a part of your cervix removed?

The risks of LEEP procedures include the discomfort of the procedure, the risk of bleeding, infection, and potential impact on future fertility. In general, the procedure is well tolerated, but injecting the numbing medicine can be uncomfortable and gives some patients a brief sense of lightheadedness. Bleeding is common but minimal, and only in rare occasions would a stitch be required. In even rarer occasions (less than 1 percent of the time), patients need to be brought to the operating room to stop the bleeding.

Infection is rare and usually is associated with a fever, pain in the pelvis, and at times, a heavy discharge. The majority of these can be treated with antibiotics taken by mouth. On extremely rare occasions, a patient may have to be admitted to a hospital to receive antibiotics through a vein for a severe infection.

A single LEEP procedure usually does not impact a woman's fertility but multiple procedures can. If a woman needs more than one LEEP procedure, precautions (as outlined in the section on cone biopsy) should be followed. Cryotherapy patients note a heavy watery discharge for a week or two after the procedure. Bleeding and infection are rare. However, a cryotherapy procedure may make it more difficult for a healthcare provider to monitor the cervix in the future, and this is one reason it is falling out of favor as a preferred technique. Laser procedures generally do not produce much pain due to the extent of anesthetic administered prior to starting. However, both infection and bleeding are rare events.

25. Are there alternatives to excision?

Alternatives to excision can be categorized as either observational or nonsurgical. There are many women for whom the best treatment of precancerous changes on their cervix is no treatment at all. This group includes those with low-grade precancerous changes (cervical intraepithelial neoplasia level I, CIN I). In young women who do not smoke, 50 percent of the precancerous changes will go away on their own, though the time for these types of changes to go away can take up to 2 years. Still, in the absence of any more severe changes during the 2-year period of observation, one can afford to be patient and allow the body's immune system to work.

Nonsurgical interventions have been looked at in the management of cervical dysplasia over the years. Beta-carotene, vitamin A derivatives, and other topical treatments have been tested. Other agents such as difloromethylomithine and indole-3-carbinol also have been evaluated. These treatments work for some women, but not for all. Unfortunately, when compared to placebo (an inactive substance), none of these therapies have proven to be effective.

Placebo

In clinical trials, it refers to the use of pills that possess no medicinal properties.

Newer studies are testing whether newer drugs or vaccines will help in women with cervical dysplasia. The Gynecologic Oncology Group of the National Cancer Institute has an ongoing clinical trial evaluating how effective a pain reliever called celecoxib is in this group of women, and a series of these types of trials is planned.

Women with cervical dysplasia should ask their healthcare providers about nonsurgical alternatives and if any are available in their area. If successful, treatment of abnormal cervical findings can become less invasive in the future.

26. Do the recommendations for treatment change if I am pregnant?

The evaluation of an abnormal Pap test in pregnancy is in many ways similar to that for nonpregnant women. Pap tests are recommended in early pregnancy, and the rate of abnormal Pap tests in pregnant women is in the vicinity of 1 to 2 percent. Colposcopy is recommended and performed in the same way and, if indicated, a biopsy is performed. However one test, called an ECC, is not performed in pregnancy because it can cause a puncture of the fetal sac and cause loss of pregnancy.

Pap tests are recommended in early pregnancy, and the rate of abnormal Pap tests in pregnant women is in the vicinity of 1 to 2 percent.

Unlike screening, the *treatment* of cervical dysplasia in the pregnant woman differs from that of the nonpregnant woman. However, the guiding principle is to do no harm to the pregnancy. With that in mind, invasive procedures, such as LEEP, laser, cryotherapy, and cold knife cone biopsies are rarely performed, unless there is a strong indication. The most commonly cited reason to do an invasive procedure in pregnancy is a strong concern that a woman has an invasive cancer.

If it is the opinion of the healthcare provider performing the colposcopy that the abnormality on the cervix is low grade in nature, a biopsy may be deferred. If a biopsy is performed, management depends on how severe of an abnormality is identified. There have been many studies focused on the management of abnormal Pap tests and abnormal cervical findings in pregnancy. The majority have shown that precancerous changes do not worsen during pregnancy and that observation is the best management until the patient delivers her baby. In many cases, the act of delivering a child can cause a strong local immune response in the cervix that may clear the changes. This has been shown to occur in as many as half of the patients in some studies.

Conservative management after the initial diagnosis for pregnant women includes repeating the colposcopic evaluation one or two more times during the pregnancy, depending on when the first one was performed. The goal of the follow-up colposcopy is to see if there have been changes in the appearance of the abnormal cervical findings that would warrant a biopsy.

For women who are suspected of having invasive cancer, the most common surgical intervention is a cone biopsy, usually performed with a scalpel as opposed to other methods such as LEEP or laser. The performance of a cone biopsy can be anxiety producing for the pregnant patient because it involves surgery close to the uterus and the developing baby. However, there have been several studies showing this is a safe procedure with only rare pregnancy loss.

PART FIVE

Diagnosis and Staging: Invasive Cervical Cancer

Are there different types of
invasive cervical cancer?

What is a prognostic indicator?
Are there indicators in cervical cancer?

How can my doctor tell if
my cancer has spread?

More . . .

27. Are there different types of invasive cervical cancer?

There are a variety of invasive cervical cancer types. The most common cancers in the cervix originate within the cervix. The cervix is a rare site to which other cancers may spread. The more common types of cancer that can spread to the cervix are cancers of the uterus or other female pelvic organs.

The type of invasive cervical cancer is defined by the type of cells seen under the microscope. This means that the best way to tell what kind of cervical cancer a woman has is to perform a biopsy.

The most common type of invasive cervical cancer is squamous cell carcinoma. Squamous cells are the cells that make up the majority of our skin lining through-out the body, including the cervix. Squamous cell car-cinomas account for approximately 75 percent of all cervical cancers. Within squamous cell carcinomas, there is one subtype that is less aggressive than the oth-ers. This type of tumor, **villoglandular carcinoma**, tends to have a growth pattern that stays on the cervix and rarely involves the surrounding tissue.

The second most common type is **adenocarcinoma,** which indicates that the cancer arose within the glands in the cervix. These glandular cells can also be found throughout the lining tissues of the body, such as the colon and breast. The cervix has a glandular lining on the inner part of the cervix next to the uterus, and this is where adenocarcinomas of the cervix arise. Adeno-carcinomas of the cervix account for approximately 20 percent of all cancers of the cervix.

Villoglandular carcinoma

A specific type of invasive cancer that typically does not spread to the surrounding tissues of the cervix. It is a less aggressive variant of cervical cancer.

Adenocarcinoma

A glandular-type of cancer that arises from different parts of the body, including the cervix.

Squamous cell carcinomas and adenocarcinomas of the cervix are associated with HPV, and testing for the virus in cancer specimens shows that almost 100 percent are positive. Stage for stage, these two types of cancers have similar rates of survival for the woman with cervical cancer.

Other cell types, which combined make up approximately 5 percent of all cancers of the cervix, include neuroendocrine carcinoma, melanoma, carcinosarcoma, serous adenocarcinoma, adenosquamous carcinoma, and lymphoma. Neuroendocrine cancers of the cervix are very aggressive. Even if diagnosed in early stage, they have a strong tendency to recur and, as a result, survival rates are lower. Women with this diagnosis tend to undergo more extensive therapy due to the aggressive nature of the cancer type. Lymphomas need to be identified because the treatment for these types of cancer differ greatly from the more common cell types.

28. What is a prognostic indicator? Are there indicators in cervical cancer?

Prognostic indicators are findings from the evaluation of a cancerous tumor that can lend some insight into the length of survival and chance of cure for the individual cancer patient. These indicators can be seen on both the clinical examination and in findings from under the microscope.

The strongest prognostic indicator in cancer of the cervix is stage (**Table 2**). The stage of a cancer is an effort to describe the extent of spread of cancer cells. As the stage at cancer diagnosis increases, the likelihood of long-term survival and possibly cure decreases. This is true for most cancers in the body.

Table 2 Staging of Cervical Cancer

Stage 0	Carcinoma in situ: Cancer-like changes noted, but without findings that the cancer has spread into the surrounding tissue (stroma).

Stage I	Cancer, confined to the cervix
	  Ia Invasive cancer with stromal invasion no more than 5 mm deep and 7 mm wide.
	    Ia1 Stromal invasion 3 mm or less in depth.
	    Ia2 Measured stromal invasion of more than 3 mm and less than 5 mm.
	  Ib The lesion on the cervix is visible on exam or shows more stromal invasion than a Ia lesion.
	    Ib1 The tumor is less than 4 cm.
	    Ib2 The tumor is greater than 4 cm.

Stage II	Cancer extends to the uterus.
	  IIa No obvious involvement of the adjacent soft tissue (parametrium).
	  IIb Obvious parametrial involvement.

Stage III	Cancer extends to involve the vagina or is causing kidney dysfunction.
	  IIIa Tumor involves the vagina.
	  IIIb Tumor extends to the pelvic wall and/or is affecting the kidney's ability to drain urine (hydronephrosis).

Stage IV	The carcinoma has extended beyond the pelvis or involves the bladder or rectum.
	  IVa Tumor invades the bladder or rectum.
	  IVb Tumor found outside of the pelvis (lungs and liver, for example).

Source: Adapted from Quinn M, Benedet JL, Odicino F, Maisonneuve P, et al. Carcinoma of the Cervix Uteri. *Internat J Gyn Onc.* 2006; 95(supp 1): S43–S103.

In general, one can break down the stages into those without spread outside of the cervix (stage I) and those that have spread either into adjacent tissues (stages II, III, and IVA) or even to more distant sites (metastases) such as the liver or lung (stage IVB). Prognostic indicators for patients with stage I cancer of the cervix include several factors. The first is tumor size. There is a definite relationship between the size of the cervical cancer and outcome. Within stage I, there is a division into IA and IB. In general, stage IA cancers can be seen

DIAGNOSIS AND STAGING: INVASIVE CERVICAL CANCER

only under the microscope, while stage IB cancers are visible and can be measured. Patients with stage IA cancer have smaller tumors and improved outcomes. Another prognostic indicator is how deeply the cervical cancer invades into the cervix. This depth of invasion has been shown to predict the risk of spread and therefore outcome. A microscopic predictor in stage I cancers is the presence of cancer cells in blood vessels or lymphatic vessels. This also can predict a more aggressive tendency. Healthcare providers use this combination of tumor size, depth of invasion, and spread into blood or lymphatic vessels to determine the type of treatment for stage I cervical cancer patients.

Another prognostic indicator is cell type. The more common types, squamous cell carcinoma and adenocarcinoma, have similar outcomes stage for stage. However, neuroendocrine carcinoma, melanoma, and possible adenosquamous carcinoma, have worse outcomes than the more common cell types even in earlier stages.

The presence of spread to distant organs (stage IVB) is an indicator of a very poor prognosis. Most treatment offered to patients diagnosed in this stage is palliative in nature with hopes of extending survival but rarely with the intent of cure.

29. How can my doctor tell if my cancer has spread?

The doctor finds the extent to which the cancer has spread by doing a staging evaluation. For women with cervical cancer, the hallmark of staging is the pelvic exam, in addition to a general physical exam. Although the pelvic exam most often is performed in your doctor's office, on occasion it must be done under anesthesia requiring an operating room. Usually this is the case if your doctor cannot fully see the cervix, if the pelvic exam causes too much pain, or if your own anatomy makes an office exam unreliable.

Along with the pelvic examination, radiology studies including a chest X-ray and an intravenous **pyelogram** (a dye test that studies the kidneys, the bladder, and the **ureters**, the drainage tubes that run from the kidneys to the bladder), a cystoscopy (looking inside the bladder with a scope), and a **proctoscopy** (looking into the anus and rectum with a scope) are done. These usually can be performed at the time of an examination under anesthesia. Although more sophisticated tests such as computed tomography (CT), magnetic resonance imaging (MRI), and fluorodeoxyglucose positron emission testing (FDG-PET) are also used, they are not a part of how we stage cervical cancer. A large part of the reason is because cervical cancer is a far larger problem in other parts of the world, especially in developing nations, where access to these modern technologies is not readily available. As a part of this international community, women's cancer specialists in gynecologic oncology are committed to a common means of staging so that all women undergo similar diagnostic procedures and results among experts in the field are communicated in a common language.

Cervical cancer staging is divided into four stages (see Table 2 on page 41). In summary, stage I cancers are those limited to the body of the cervix with no evidence of spread. Stage IA cancers are evident only at the microscopic level, while stage IB cancers are either visible with the naked eye or have evidence of more advanced

Pyelogram

A radiologic test that specifically looks at the kidney and ureters.

Ureters

Tubes that connect the kidneys to the bladder for passing urine.

Proctoscopy

A technique using a scope to examine the rectum, anus, and colon.

Cervical cancer staging is divided into four stages.

43

Parametria

The connective tissue and fat that lies adjacent to the uterus.

spread under the microscope. Stage II cancers of the cervix have spread outside of the cervix to the nearby soft tissue (**parametria**) or cardinal ligament but have not reached the sidewall of the pelvis. Stage III cancers have more advanced local spread. Stage IIIA cancers include those that have spread to the lower part of the vagina. Stage IIIB cancers of the cervix demonstrate spread out to the sidewall of the pelvis, either identified as such on pelvic exam or by the finding of blockage of the ureter (hydronephrosis or hydroureter) on imaging tests. Stage IV tumors have two distinct subsets. Stage IVA tumors have more locally advanced spread to the lining of the bladder or rectum. Stage IVB tumors have distant spread or metastases.

30. What is a PET scan? Does it play a role in cervical cancer?

Positron emission test (PET) scan

A radiologic test that uses information on the metabolism of cells to differentiate normal from abnormal tissue. Highly active tissue on a PET scan in a patient with cervical cancer can indicate that cancer has spread to that area.

CT scans

Computed tomography scans used as a diagnostic imaging test.

As mentioned above, an **FDG-PET (fluorodeoxyglucose positron emission test) scan** is a radiologic study that uses information about the metabolism or activity of tumors to determine the extent a cancer has spread. A PET scan is done by labeling glucose (or sugar) molecules with a radioactive tag and then scanning for where these molecules show up in the body. Highly metabolic or active spots are suspicious for being cancerous, although there are areas, such as the kidney or bladder, that routinely show activity as well.

Oftentimes, PET scans are combined with **CT scans** to help give both a structural and functional assessment of a tumor. For instance, an area of activity on a PET scan appears as a blurry area on the outline of your body. Adding a CT scan allows your doctor to locate the area on a PET scan to see if there is a growth or tumor that corresponds to that activity.

44

The role of PET scanning in cervical cancer is becoming more and more popular in industrialized countries. It can determine if there are sites of activity outside of the pelvis, which is helpful in determining whether a patient is a candidate to receive radiation therapy to the pelvis. PET scans also can help decide whether a patient has responded well to her combined chemotherapy and radiation. PET scans performed after completion of primary therapy can give a good sense of whether a patient may be cured of her disease. However, this aspect of PET scans is still in the research phase. In addition, PET scans can help in follow-ups. For example, if a CT scan done long after treatment has been completed is "suspicious," then a PET scan can tell if there is activity in the area—a finding that may point toward a cancer recurrence. In other words, PET scans can be done to see if your cancer has become metastatic or has recurred. There are ongoing studies looking at the role of PET scans in cervical cancer and other gynecologic cancers. Overtime, this is likely to be a well-accepted and frequently performed test for women with cancer of the cervix.

The role of PET scanning in cervical cancer is becoming more and more popular in industrialized countries.

31. How does cervical cancer spread?

Cancer of the cervix initially spreads locally first, which explains the way it is staged. The cancer starts in the cervix and then spreads out to the sides of the pelvis through the support structure of the cervix and uterus called the **cardinal ligament**. The cancer then can attach to the walls of the pelvis. Cancer of the cervix also can spread toward the front of the cervix and into the bladder or out the back of the cervix into the rectum. Spread to the bladder or rectum is not as common as spread toward the side of the pelvis.

cardinal ligament
A fibrous band attached to the cervix and the vagina laterally, extending to the uterus, to provide support. It also contains the blood vessels to the pelvis.

DIAGNOSIS AND STAGING: INVASIVE CERVICAL CANCER

45

Lymphatic spread also occurs in cervical cancer but not as commonly. Sometimes, patients who are thought to have cancer confined to the cervix are found to have lymph node spread at the time of surgery. This finding can have a significant impact on how doctors treat the cervical cancer patient, especially as it relates to decisions about surgery versus no surgery, radiation or no radiation. Another situation that demonstrates this type of spread involves patients who have cancer spread within their pelvis but on CT scan are found to have lymph node involvement higher up in the abdomen or chest separate from the primary tumor. This finding may lead to a change in the primary approach of treatment to take into account the extent of spread.

There are three lymph node regions in the body that are important in the management of cancer of the cervix.

Hematogenous spread can occur as well but is usually a sign of very advanced disease. Common sites for this type of spread are the lungs or liver. Unfortunately, this type of spread is a very bad sign for a woman with cancer of the cervix.

32. How do I know if my lymph nodes are involved?

Determining if the **lymph nodes** are involved is very important for patients with cancer of the cervix. Decisions regarding treatment are often based on the presence or absence of tumor within the lymph nodes.

Lymph nodes

A part of the lymphatic system, these are glands composed of lymphocytes that act as the filtration system of the body.

Pelvic lymph nodes

A group of nodes that lie within the pelvis. These are at high risk of being involved with cervical cancer.

There are three lymph node regions in the body that are important in the management of cancer of the cervix. The first are the **pelvic lymph nodes**. The pelvic lymph nodes exist in chains that run alongside blood vessels and are found along both sides of the pelvis. The extent of the pelvic lymph nodes ends at the top of the pelvis.

The second lymph node region is called the **para-aortic area**. These are lymph nodes just above the top of the pelvis that are adjacent to the main blood vessels that connect to the lower part of the body, specifically the aorta and vena cava. The third region of lymph nodes includes those that are not in the pelvic or para-aortic area.

The status of the pelvic lymph nodes is most crucial in determining therapy for early stage cervical cancer patients. The surgery for women with early stage cervical cancer includes a radical or extended hysterectomy and dissection of the pelvic lymph nodes. If the pelvic lymph nodes are involved, the patient is at a higher risk of recurrence, and radiation therapy combined with chemotherapy is administered after surgery. Knowing the status of the para-aortic lymph nodes at this time is important as well. If the para-aortic lymph nodes are not involved in a patient with pelvic lymph node spread, then the radiation field can be focused on the pelvis alone. In more advanced cancer of the cervix with spread inside the pelvis, patients commonly do not undergo surgery. These patients usually are treated with a stronger type of radiation along with chemotherapy.

There are multiple ways a surgeon can determine if lymph nodes are involved in cervical cancer. The first is at the time of surgery—when the lymph nodes are removed at the time of the hysterectomy. The second method is by doing a biopsy with a needle. The health-care provider performing the needle biopsy is usually aided by radiology. Using a CT scan machine, the needle can be guided to the suspicious area. The third technique is combining a CT scan and a PET scan, known as a PET/CT scan. In this combined scan, abnormal active areas are correlated with areas that are

Para-aortic area

The region near the aorta; it generally refers to a group of nodes that can be involved by cancer of the cervix.

also enlarged, and if both are present in the lymph nodes in a woman with cervical cancer, it is considered proof of metastatic disease. In such a case, your doctor may not even proceed to a biopsy or excision.

33. What is a sentinel node biopsy?

The lymph nodes, or glands, within the pelvis and lower abdominal area can be affected in women with cervical cancer. A cancer that has spread to the lymph nodes generally requires more aggressive treatment and is associated with a poorer prognosis.

Lymphocele

A sac of lymph fluid usually as the result of surgery and/or damage to the lymphatic system.

However, removal of lymph nodes is not without potential complications. At the time of surgery, removing lymph nodes adds time to the surgery and can be associated with a risk of bleeding. Fluid collections, called **lymphoceles**, can occur after surgery. In the long term, some patients may experience swelling of the legs, or **lymphedema**.

Lymphedema

The backup of lymph fluid due to an obstruction or the removal of lymph nodes that results in the swelling of the affected body part.

In an effort to decrease these complications while at the same time obtaining the information necessary to make appropriate treatment decisions, the process of **sentinel lymph node biopsies** is being evaluated in women with cervical cancer. This process, which attempts to identify the lymph node at highest risk, has been evaluated in breast cancer. In theory, removing less lymph nodes should lead to less complications, such as arm swelling or lymphedema. Based on many large studies, sentinel lymph node biopsy is now performed in place of a full lymph node dissection in women with breast cancer.

Sentinel lymph node biopsy

A technique using dye and/or a radioactive substance injected into the tumor with the aim of identifying its drainage pattern in the lymph system. The first node(s) that are identified are termed the sentinel node.

The technique of sentinel node biopsy in cervical cancer requires two different injections into the cervix before surgery. One injection is a radioisotope, Technetium-

99, which can be tracked with a Geiger counter–type instrument. The other injection is a colored dye of which there are several types. Upon opening the abdomen at the time of surgery, the leading lymph nodes are identified either by their radioactivity, their color, or both. These lymph nodes are then removed and analyzed.

However, in cervical cancer, the performance of a sentinel lymph node biopsy has not yet been adopted as a standard of care. Studies are ongoing to determine if the sentinel lymph nodes accurately predict what is going on in the rest of the lymph nodes and if the survival of women with cervical cancer is affected. If you have cancer of the cervix and are undergoing surgery, ask your surgeon about this technique and the opportunity to participate in important studies involving sentinel lymph node dissection.

If you have cancer of the cervix and are undergoing surgery, ask your surgeon about this technique and the opportunity to participate in important studies involving sentinel lymph node dissection.

DIAGNOSIS AND STAGING: INVASIVE CERVICAL CANCER

PART SIX

Treatment of Invasive Cervical Cancer: Early-Stage Disease

What does it mean to have early invasive cervical cancer?

How is early cervical cancer treated?

Are there surgical options if I want to have children in the future?

More . . .

34. What does it mean to have early invasive cervical cancer?

If you are diagnosed with cervical cancer, one of the first priorities is to determine the stage of the cancer. The process of diagnosing an early invasive cervical cancer involves multiple steps. The first step is the evaluation of the abnormal Pap test. This requires a colposcopy, a microscopic evaluation of the cervix. Using the visibility provided by the colposcope, the appropriate area for biopsy can best be determined. Some women with early invasive cervical cancer have only a severely precancerous biopsy, while others may show some evidence of or suspicion for an invasive cervical cancer.

The performance of a cone biopsy, discussed at length in Question 22, is critical for deciding whether a cervical cancer is an early, or **microinvasive**, cancer or more advanced. The cone biopsy is sectioned, or cut, into multiple specimens to allow for thorough analysis by the pathologist to determine if there is invasion. Cervical cancers that invade less than 5 millimeters ($\frac{1}{5}$th of an inch) into the wall of the cervix and spread less than 7 millimeters ($\frac{3}{10}$th of an inch) in width qualify as microinvasive cancer of the cervix.

Being diagnosed with early cervical cancer means that a woman may need further treatment beyond her cone biopsy. The type and extent of treatment depend on the patient's age, desire for fertility, and status of the margins on the cone biopsy. Older patients usually opt for a hysterectomy, while younger women may wish to be more conservative due to fertility desires. A cone biopsy with a positive or involved margin may require a repeat cone biopsy or may indicate the need for more aggressive therapy.

Microinvasive

In cervical cancer, it refers to the microscopic finding of cancer cells that have penetrated the usual border in small collections. It represents the earliest evidence of invasion.

TREATMENT OF INVASIVE CERVICAL CANCER: EARLY-STAGE DISEASE

35. How is early cervical cancer treated?

Early, or microinvasive, cervical cancer is treated based on several factors. The first factor is the extent of the cancer in the cone biopsy. For very early cancers, a simple hysterectomy can be a curative procedure. For early cancers that have more extensive depth of invasion, or **roots**, into the surrounding cervical tissues, a more extended or radical hysterectomy may be indicated. The standard of care in regards to how deep is deep enough to require radical surgery differs in different institutions and countries.

In some centers, a cone biopsy with negative margins is considered sufficient for very early cervical cancer, whereas others may recommend a hysterectomy. Other factors that are evaluated by the pathologist in diagnosing are vascular space, or blood vessel, invasion and lymphatic space (channels that carry lymph fluid through the body) invasion. The presence of invasion in these spaces can indicate a higher risk of spread for patients with very early cervical cancer. In patients who have lymphatic or vascular space invasion, a hysterectomy may be the preferred option.

The second and third factors are age and desire for fertility. These generally go together because postmenopausal women and women who have completed having children tend to be older than women who have not yet had children or were planning further childbearing. In women who desire giving birth in the future after their cervical cancer diagnosis, a cone biopsy would retain fertility if they had an early invasive cervical cancer. In women who have completed or otherwise do not desire future childbearing, a hysterectomy is generally the preferred option. However, even in patients who desire fu-

Roots

The finding that cancer has involved deeper into normal tissue or extended outside the place it started.

ture fertility, caution must be exercised in being too conservative, especially if findings in the original cancer diagnosis suggest a high risk of recurrence.

36. Are there surgical options if I want to have children in the future?

Yes, there are surgical options for women with early stage cervical cancer if they want to have children in the future. However, the available options depend on the size and stage of the cervical cancer. Also of critical importance is evaluating the patient with computed tomography (CT) scans to make certain that there is no evidence of cancer outside of the cervix.

For a woman with a very early invasive cancer of the cervix, a cone biopsy may be sufficient treatment for her cancer. This is true if the depth of invasion, or roots, of the cancer are minimal. The absence of any invasion into the vascular or lymphatic spaces is also important for this strategy.

Radical trachelectomy is an option for a woman with a diagnosis of cervical cancer who wishes to retain her childbearing capabilities. Radical trachelectomy is a surgical procedure that involves removing the cervix and surrounding tissues usually in combination with removal of the pelvic lymph nodes. This technique has been developed and evaluated over the past 10 to 20 years and has been found to be a relatively safe and effective procedure for women who wish to retain their uterus. For women with very early cervical cancer with risk factors, such as deeply invasive disease or when it is visible to the naked eye but still limited to the cervix, radical trachelectomy is the most appropriate option for

Radical trachelectomy

A surgical procedure for early cervical cancer that involves removing the cervix only. It is a technique that allows women to maintain the potential of carrying a pregnancy.

55

a women who wishes to keep her uterus. At the time of a radical trachelectomy, a supportive suture must be placed in the base of the uterus in an attempt to strengthen the lower part of the uterus. Because the cervix is removed, there is nothing to prevent early pregnancy loss. Women who select this option must be cautioned that future pregnancy is high risk in nature. In studies, many of the women who became pregnant after radical trachelectomy experienced premature deliveries due to the absence of the cervix.

The option for a woman who has to have her uterus and cervix removed for cervical cancer is surrogate motherhood. The ovaries do not have to be removed as part of radical surgery for cervical cancer. Afterwards, assisted reproductive technologies can be performed to stimulate egg growth in the ovaries. These eggs can be removed and fertilized outside of the body and implanted in a surrogate carrier.

37. How does a surgeon decide if I can keep my uterus?

In the case of a woman who is going to have fertility-sparing surgery for her early stage cervical cancer, the decision to keep the uterus is dependent on several factors. Those factors are determined before, during, or after surgery.

Prior to undergoing a fertility-sparing surgery, a CT scan generally is performed to evaluate for the possibility of spread outside of the cervix. If there is evidence of spread to a lymph node, fertility-sparing surgery that would allow a woman to keep her uterus would not be performed. If there is evidence of spread outside of the cervix, radiation is administered after or in place of surgery. Radiation therapy makes future childbearing impossible.

At the time of a fertility-sparing surgery such as a radical trachelectomy, the surgeon will look to see if there is evidence of spread outside of the cervix. The places of concern include the lymph nodes and the areas next to the cervix. If there is evidence of cancer in the lymph nodes or in the tissue next to the cervix, the operation may be converted to removal of the uterus as well as the cervix. After surgery, it is likely that radiation will be required.

Sometimes, after surgery, the final pathology findings will demonstrate evidence of cancer in the lymph nodes or in the tissues next to the cervix that were not otherwise visible at the time of surgery. Unfortunately, these findings indicate the need for additional treatment after surgery such as radiation and/or chemotherapy.

38. What if I don't want surgery? What other options do I have?

If you do not want surgery for your diagnosis of cervical cancer, there may be other options that offer you a similar outcome to surgery. This is mainly true for women with a diagnosis of early stage cervical cancer.

Radiation therapy has been used for women with cervical cancer since the early 1900s. Historically, radiation therapy has been associated with a variety of side effects. Over the years, radiation techniques have improved greatly with the development of linear accelerators. As the medical profession's ability to increase the power of the radiation has improved, the side effects associated with this treatment have decreased.

Radiation therapy has been used for women with cervical cancer since the early 1900s.

TREATMENT OF INVASIVE CERVICAL CANCER: EARLY-STAGE DISEASE

Women who do not wish to have surgery for their diagnosis of cervical cancer may be offered treatment with radiation therapy, generally in combination with chemotherapy as primary treatment. The treatment with radiation therapy usually lasts about 8 weeks. The first 5 to 6 weeks involves daily external radiation treatments from a linear accelerator that last only a few minutes each day. Chemotherapy is given one time per week during the external treatments. At the conclusion of the external treatments, or sometimes during the treatments, another form of radiation, **brachytherapy**, is administered. Brachytherapy is usually given in two long doses or five short doses. Brachytherapy is performed by bringing the radiation source directly to the cervix through a temporary catheter inserted into the vagina.

Brachytherapy

The technique of giving radiation by placing the radioactive source directly inside or next to the area of treatment. In cervical cancer, the source generally is placed inside the vagina so that the cervix can be treated specifically.

39. What does it mean to have stage IB cervical cancer? Is it still curable?

Stage IB cervical cancer is still considered an early stage of cervical cancer. These cancers can span from the barely visible to tumors that are 1 to 2 inches across. As the tumors increase in size, the chances that the cancer will have left the cervix and spread elsewhere increase. Most women with stage IB cervical cancer are treated with surgery alone, although 15 to 20 percent of patients will need additional therapy after surgery such as radiation. Fortunately, most women who have stage IB cervical cancer will be cured of their disease.

40. Are stage IB tumors treated differently than other early cervical cancers?

Because stage IB cervical cancers include such a wide array of tumor sizes, not even all stage IB cervical cancers are treated the same. For patients with very large stage IB cervical cancers (those that are in excess of 4 centimeters), there is no consensus. Many healthcare providers prefer the use of radiation therapy with chemotherapy as the primary mode of treatment. Their rationale is that 30 to 40 percent of women who have surgery for a tumor of this size will need radiation therapy after surgery anyway. Others believe there is still a benefit to surgery regardless of the need for radiation therapy for those women who have findings at surgery that need additional treatment.

In very small stage IB cervical cancers, there is a general consensus among healthcare providers that surgery is the preferred route, unless the patient has other health concerns that may make surgery dangerous.

41. Do the treatment recommendations change if I am pregnant?

The treatment recommendations for cervical cancer are based on the stage of the disease and the overall health of the patient. Women with cervical cancer who are pregnant unfortunately face the very difficult decision of whether to keep the pregnancy.

When a woman who is pregnant is diagnosed with cervical cancer, the first step is to determine how far along she is in her pregnancy. For women who are near the date of delivery, their cancer treatment can be deferred until after she delivers. Patients who are diagnosed earlier in pregnancy need to decide what to do with the pregnancy for two main reasons. The first is that either accepted treatment for early stage cervical cancer, be it surgery or radiation, is fatal to the developing fetus. The second reason is that delay in treatment may lead to progression of the cervical cancer and possibly a worse outcome for the patient.

TREATMENT OF INVASIVE CERVICAL CANCER: EARLY-STAGE DISEASE

Some women choose to keep their pregnancy despite a diagnosis of cervical cancer even in the early stages of pregnancy. If a woman's cervical cancer is very early stage, such as microinvasive, the risk of progression in pregnancy is small, and once delivery occurs, immediate therapy usually results in a favorable outcome. Cervical cancers that can be seen or felt on exam need to be watched more carefully. If no growth is evident, therapy for the cancer should be performed as soon as the baby is mature and can be safely delivered, usually before the expected due date. For some cancers that are more advanced or that grow during the pregnancy, chemotherapy has been administered in an attempt to keep the cancer under control until the baby can be safely delivered.

PART SEVEN

Treatment of Invasive Cervical Cancer: Locally Advanced Disease

What does it mean if my cancer
is locally advanced?

Shouldn't surgery still be done if my cancer
has spread beyond my cervix?

What is the standard of care for treatment
for locally advanced cervical cancer?

More . . .

42. What does it mean if my cancer is locally advanced?

A cancer of the cervix is considered locally advanced if it has spread outside of the cervix. Common sites of spread for locally advanced cervical cancer include the vagina, the parametria (the soft tissues next to the cervix), and the bony sidewall of the pelvis. Less-common sites of local spread include the bladder and rectum. Spread to any of these sites results in a stage II or greater stage cancer diagnosis.

A cancer of the cervix is considered locally advanced if it has spread outside of the cervix.

When planning treatment for a woman with locally advanced cervical cancer, further radiologic tests are important. A computed tomography (CT) scan or other radiologic test can define whether a locally advanced cervical cancer on exam has spread outside of the pelvis. If a locally advanced cervical cancer has not spread outside of the pelvis, aggressive treatment with a combination of radiation and chemotherapy can result in a cure for many of these women.

43. Shouldn't surgery still be done if my cancer has spread beyond my cervix?

It would seem to make sense that if a cancer of the cervix can be safely removed surgically, this option should be offered to women even with locally advanced disease. However, this is not true. It has been shown that performing surgery on most women with locally advanced cervical cancer actually results in a worse prognosis. If they undergo surgery as opposed to primary radiation with chemotherapy for locally advanced cervical cancer and a portion of the cancer is left inside the patient, treatment calls for the use of radiation. However, when the cervix is absent, only external beam radiation can be delivered, and this may be insufficient to treat the remaining cancer. Usually, to treat cervical cancer with a hope for cure, a combination of external and internal radiation, where radiation implants are placed onto the cervix directly, is required. Because the cervix is removed at the time of surgery, this cannot be done and inadequate treatment with a worse prognosis may be the result.

44. What is the standard of care for treatment for locally advanced cervical cancer?

Locally advanced cervical cancer means that the cancer has left the cervix and spread to adjacent tissues or organs in the pelvis. The standard of care treatment for locally advanced cervical cancer is a combination of radiation therapy and chemotherapy. The radiation therapy is given in two parts. The first part is a series of external treatments, much like shining a beam of light, to the pelvic area of a woman with cervical cancer. Before the start of treatment, a sophisticated set of measurements is performed through a combination of CT scan imaging and calculations involving the physical properties of radiation. These calculations are performed by the radiation doctor and scientists called radiation physicists. The external treatments are administered daily over 25 to 28 days.

Locally advanced cervical cancer means that the cancer has left the cervix and spread to adjacent tissues or organs in the pelvis.

Either during or after the external treatments, internal treatments called brachytherapy are done. Brachytherapy means bringing the radioactive source directly to the tumor. In cervical cancer patients, this is accomplished by placement of a narrow tube, called a **tandem**, through the vagina and into the cervix. The advantage of the brachytherapy is that higher radiation doses can

Tandem

In radiation, it is the tube that is inserted into the vagina to allow direct radiation of the cervix.

be brought directly to the tumor without causing undue damage to the tissues and organs surrounding the cervix.

In 1999, the National Cancer Institute, based on a series of five pivotal studies, concluded that the addition of a weekly chemotherapy treatment improved the outcome for women with locally advanced cervical cancer. A drug called cisplatin is the most common chemotherapy agent used in this situation. It is given through a vein over 1 to 2 hours one time per week. The chemotherapy treatment is usually well tolerated and does not cause hair loss like some other chemotherapy agents.

45. What is neoadjuvant chemotherapy?

Neoadjuvant chemotherapy is the use of chemotherapy to help reduce the size of a cancer with the hopes of eventually performing surgery to get rid of the cancer that remains. In patients with stage IB2 cervical cancer (localized to the cervix but greater than 4 centimeters in size), neoadjuvant chemotherapy could be used to shrink the size of the tumor, hopefully reducing the extent of surgery that needs to be performed. There has been one large study in the United States evaluating this concept, but unfortunately that program closed early and the question remains unanswered. In Europe and Asia, the concept of neoadjuvant chemotherapy is being evaluated for more locally advanced cervical cancers with the hope of shrinking them to allow for complete surgical resection. This will be effective only if the cervical cancer can be reduced in size to allow complete resection. Anything less than complete removal of the tumor may worsen the prognosis for cervical cancer patients.

Neoadjuvant chemotherapy

The use of cancer drugs as first treatment aimed at reducing the size or involvement of cancer.

Based on the lack of conclusive evidence supporting its use, neoadjuvant chemotherapy is rarely used in cervical cancer.

46. What if I am pregnant? Can I wait until after I have my baby to be treated?

At the time of a cervical cancer diagnosis, some women may be pregnant. The recommendations for treatment of cervical cancer do not change if a woman is pregnant. Treatment should consist of standard-of-care recommendations based on the stage of disease. In the case of pregnancy, a woman may opt to postpone definitive treatment until after delivery but must be aware of the risk of the cancer getting worse during that time. If a woman is diagnosed with locally advanced disease, termination of pregnancy may be required to save her life. This difficult discussion of the risks to your health, the benefits of intervening now while you are pregnant, and your desire to keep the pregnancy must be honestly and openly discussed with your doctor.

PART EIGHT

Treatment of Metastatic, Advanced, or Recurrent Cervical Cancer

What is the prognosis for women
whose disease is advanced?

How can cervical cancer come back
if my cervix was removed?

What is a pelvic exenteration?
Who should be considered for this?

More . . .

47. What is the prognosis for women whose disease is advanced?

Similar to most cancers, the prognosis for women with cervical cancer is mainly dependent on the stage of disease at the time of presentation. Advanced cancers of the cervix can be divided into those that are locally advanced (stage II, III, and IVA) and those that are advanced with metastases outside of the pelvis (stage IVB).

For locally advanced cervical cancer, the prognosis is based on the stage of disease. For stage II disease, about 60 percent will be cured of their cancer, representing the majority of women diagnosed at this stage. For stage III disease, the cure rate falls to 30 to 40 percent and for women with stage IVA disease, the prognosis is even more guarded.

Women who are diagnosed with a stage IVB cervical cancer, or ones with metastatic disease (spread to distant sites such as the lung or liver), are unfortunately rarely ever cured of their disease. Treatment in this setting usually is directed at the relief of symptoms (**palliation**). Sometimes, radiation may be offered to control the vaginal bleeding associated with cervical cancer. In women who do not have significant bleeding, chemotherapy may be administered.

The goal of chemotherapy in this setting is not to cure the disease but to reduce symptoms and hopefully gain temporary shrinkage of the tumor and extend the life of a patient with advanced, metastatic cervical cancer for as long as possible.

Similar to most cancers, the prognosis for women with cervical cancer is mainly dependent on the stage of disease at the time of presentation.

Palliation
To provide comfort.

48. How can cervical cancer come back if my cervix was removed?

Cancers are generally named for the organ or tissue where the cancer started. For example, if a patient is diagnosed with a colon cancer and has a nodule in the liver that contains colon cancer cells, that is metastatic disease and the nodule is called a metastasis. The metastatic nodule in the liver, however, is not called "liver" cancer.

Recurrence

Cancer that has returned despite treatment.

Remission

A designation of being cancer free.

In patients with cervical cancer, the disease may return (a **recurrence**) after a period without any evidence of the cancer (**remission**). The cells that grow back in another part of the body were likely there all along but undetectable by physical exam or X-ray. If a biopsy of the cells were performed, they would look identical underneath the microscope to the original cancer cells from the cervix and would be referred to as recurrent cervical cancer.

Darlene's comment:

About a year after my hysterectomy, I had a reoccurrence, and I had to have an anterior exenteration.

Pelvic exenteration

A radical surgical procedure that involves removal of the pelvic organs, which may include the bladder (anterior exenteration) and/or the rectum and anus (posterior exenteration). It is performed as a curative procedure in women with recurrent cervical cancer.

49. What is a pelvic exenteration? Who should be considered for this?

A **pelvic exenteration** is a very radical, or aggressive, surgical procedure intended to cure a cervical cancer patient of recurrent or persistent disease in the pelvis. The operation includes removal of the last part of the colon called the rectum, the bladder, the uterus and cervix, fallopian tubes and ovaries, and the vagina. Removing all of these organs is called a *total pelvic exenteration.*

Sometimes, if the cancer permits, the rectum may be left in place. This procedure is called an *anterior pelvic exenteration*. At other times, the bladder is left in place; this is called a *posterior pelvic exenteration*. Removing these organs then requires some alternative method of moving the bowels and urinating. For bowel function, a **colostomy** (bag) procedure is performed. In rare occasions, the bowel can be reconnected. For the urinary tract, a bag can be placed, called a **urostomy**. Sometimes, a new bladder is created out of small and large intestine that can be drained intermittently with a catheter, and the patient does not have to wear a bag for the flow of urine.

Colostomy

A surgical procedure in which a part of the colon is connected to the anterior abdominal wall. The opening of the colostomy at the wall is termed a stoma and is the means by which stool is passed.

Urostomy

An artificial opening that allows urine to pass. It is created surgically if a person needs to have the bladder removed during an exenteration.

A candidate for this procedure is usually a cervical cancer patient who has had recurrence of her disease in the center of the pelvis, either at the top of the vagina or in the cervix for patients who were treated primarily with radiation. Sometimes, a patient may have had an incomplete response to radiation therapy and is left with disease in the center of the pelvis. A thorough search for evidence of cancer outside the center of the pelvis is mandatory. Patients with recurrent cancer outside of the pelvis are not considered curable and are not offered the procedure. The complexity of and possible postoperative complications associated with this procedure make it appropriate only for a small percentage of patients with persistent or recurrent cervical cancer. Approximately one half of all patients who undergo this procedure die of their cancer despite the exhaustive preoperative search for spread outside of the pelvis.

Darlene's comment:

I didn't have my rectum removed. A neobladder was made from my intestine and now I self-catheterize through my umbilicus! My plumbing may be different, but it still works. No need to put the seat down for me!

50. What treatments are available for women whose disease is not curable?

Treatments for women whose cervical cancer is not curable depend on the symptoms they have and their overall medical condition. In an otherwise healthy woman with incurable cervical cancer, aggressive combination chemotherapy may be administered in the hopes of gaining a temporary time without evidence of her cancer (remission) or at least delaying further growth of her cancer. Elderly patients, or those with other significant medical illnesses, may not be able to tolerate such therapy.

Some patients with incurable cervical cancer still have a large amount of cancer in the pelvis, which can cause heavy vaginal bleeding or pain. The pain may come from the cancer itself or may be a result of the cancer pressing on nerves and other vital structures in the pelvis. In this setting, radiation treatments are offered to the patient in the hopes of controlling these symptoms. Some patients who have sites of the disease outside of the pelvis that cause symptoms may be offered targeted radiation to these areas as well for relief of symptoms.

Best supportive care

A treatment principle concentrated on the relief of symptoms from a disease, as opposed to treating the disease itself.

Some women with incurable cervical cancer may be best treated with no treatment at all, a concept referred to as "**best supportive care.**" Patients "treated" in this fashion receive medications for pain or other symptoms that arise but do not receive radiation therapy or chemotherapy. This is generally done in the setting of hospice care.

51. Is there a standard of care for treating metastatic cervical cancer?

There is no standard of care for treating mestastatic cervical cancer. Options exist for chemotherapy, radiation therapy, or best supportive care (see **Question 50**). In this setting, strong consideration should be given to participation in clinical trials. Response rates for conventional chemotherapy agents in this setting are usually low. The hopes of patients diagnosed with metastatic cervical cancer rest on the development of new chemotherapy agents or newer "**biologic modifiers.**"

Cancer cells grow because they have internal defects in how they control their growth. Healthy cells in a human body will self destruct once their usual life span is complete or will not divide and grow unless the circumstances are appropriate. In this setting, the healthy cells respond to signals from the body. Cancer cells do not respond to the usual signals in the body and have lost their ability to regulate their growth. The reasons for this loss of control are many and are based on the biology of the cell. Repairing or restricting these mechanisms in the cancer cells is the goal of biologic modifiers.

Biologic modifiers
Drugs or compounds that aim to stimulate or to restore the ability of the immune system to fight disease or infections.

Cancer cells grow because they have internal defects in how they control their growth.

PART NINE

Treatment at the End of Life

How will I know when I am terminal?

What does palliative care mean?

What do I tell my family?

More . . .

52. How will I know when I am terminal?

Predicting when someone enters the final phase is very difficult, but there are certain signs that are present that can help you and your doctor determine this. If you have been through a number of treatments and the cancer continues to grow or does not otherwise respond to treatment, it is not likely that further treatment will help. In addition, if pain increases, weakness worsens, or you are not able to eat, all of these are worrisome signs that the cancer cannot be medically controlled. More importantly, however, the acknowledgment that you are entering a terminal phase in your care requires an open relationship paved in honesty and trust between you and your doctor.

53. What does palliative care mean?

Palliative care is the active management of patients at the end of life. With palliative care, death is not viewed as something to be avoided, but is embraced as a part of the normal cycle of life. The aim of care at this phase is to help those who are sick remain as active as possible for as long as possible. It also is designed to manage the symptoms that can be present when a woman is at the end of her life, including active management of pain, nausea and vomiting, and tiredness. Even more than this, it is meant to address all of the issues that can accompany the end of life, including issues related to religion, fear, depression, and the other psychological and spiritual aspects of care. Finally, palliative care embraces the family and social supports of the woman with end-stage cervical cancer to assist them as they help their loved one and to help them cope in what is often a very difficult time.

TREATMENT AT THE END OF LIFE

Palliative care
A healthcare model for which attention to symptoms is as important as (or may even replace) the treatment of the disease itself.

54. What do I tell my family?

Your family and friends can be the source of strength and support for you. It is important that you allow them to help you if it is offered because no one should go through cancer alone. Part of this is keeping them as involved as you feel comfortable and letting them know where you are in your cancer journey. If things do not look good and the cancer appears to be "taking over," your support system can help you adjust to emotionally and physically hard times. Many doctors recommend appropriate honesty to their patients, encouraging them to let those who love them (and they in turn love) participate in their care as much as they are willing to, and as much as they want them to.

55. What is a living will?

Living will

A legal document that specifies a person's advance wishes in case the person is not able to consent to (or refuse) treatment. It is also known as an advance directive.

A **living will** is a legal document that covers the types of treatment you wish for yourself. It includes instructions that can be followed by your doctors and caregivers if you are not able to participate in your care. It can encompass directions related to intensive care, artificial nutrition, the use of intravenous fluids, and artificial life support. It usually is accompanied by orders regarding resuscitation and that of your healthcare proxy.

56. What does hospice mean?

Hospice

A philosophy for care at the end of life, aiming to provide patients with comfort, dignity, and quality in the last phases of an illness.

Hospice is otherwise termed end-of-life care. When treatments are no longer working and a woman becomes very sick because of her cancer, her doctor may recommend hospice. It represents a concerted effort by doctors and other healthcare providers to recognize that the end of life is a part of the disease process. Medical professionals have a responsibility to help the patient and her family remain as comfortable as possible, with dignity and free of pain. Hospice care can be delivered either in an inpatient facility (either a hospital or nursing home–type setting) or at home. The overarching goal of hospice is to ensure that women with end-stage cervical cancer die with dignity and in peace. It should not be taken to mean that your physicians are "giving up" on you. Instead, it should be viewed as an acknowledgment that a patient is entering the final phase of her life, and instead of active treatment, active care is undertaken aimed at improving each hour and each day for her and her loved ones.

The overarching goal of hospice is to ensure that women with end-stage cervical cancer die with dignity and in peace.

57. What is a DNR order?

DNR stands for "do not resuscitate." This order represents your wishes in case something happens to you that, without the use of machines, would result in your death. If you are unable to speak for yourself, these wishes will help your family, your physician, or your healthcare proxy to make decisions for you when that time comes. In a **DNR order**, you would be asked to state specifically what you would want done and what you would not want done if you were to have a life-threatening event.

DNR order

A "Do Not Resuscitate" order, which communicates a person's wishes not to be revived or kept alive through artificial means.

These decisions are in large part state determined. For example, in Connecticut, a DNR order must specify clearly if you do or do not want to have a tube inserted into your throat to help you breathe (intubation), cardiac resuscitation, intravenous fluids, or total parenteral nutrition. In New York, both intubation and cardiac resuscitation are included in the DNR order.

You should not wait to establish a DNR order until you become so sick that you have to make the decision without having time to really think about it or you are considered terminal. The best time to discuss it is when you are still healthy, so that you and your family can ask questions and thoroughly talk it over with your doctor.

It's important to realize that a DNR order is not permanent. If at any point you change your mind regarding what you would want for yourself in a life-threatening situation, your healthcare team and your family must respect your wishes.

58. What is a healthcare proxy?

Healthcare proxy

Also known as a durable power of attorney for healthcare, it is a legally named person who is tasked with making medical decisions for a person if that person is unable to make them.

If you don't designate a healthcare proxy, your family often has to make decisions for you.

A **healthcare proxy** is a person designated to make healthcare decisions for you in the event that you are unable to tell your physicians your wishes. This can be a very important role, so it's important for you as a patient to initiate a discussion of what you would want for yourself. Only then can your physicians make sure that they're abiding by your wishes. If you don't designate a healthcare proxy, your family often has to make decisions for you. Doing that can be risky because, although they may be acting with your best interests at heart, their decisions may not necessarily be what you would want. In addition, it's not uncommon for different members of your family to disagree with each other, particularly when it comes to someone they love. By designating a healthcare proxy, your family and loved ones would know that you specifically chose someone to speak for you.

PART TEN

Survivorship Issues After Cervical Cancer

What is survivorship medicine?

Now that I have had cervical cancer,
what do I do?

How are women followed after
treatment for cervical cancer?

More . . .

59. What is survivorship medicine?

Survivorship medicine is a field devoted to people who have been diagnosed and treated for cancer. The specific goals survivorship medicine encompass are prevention and early detection. In addition, it offers support of cancer families to help minimize pain, disability, and psychosocial stressors while promoting and encouraging improved quality of life for the cancer patient. The ultimate aim is to provide you, with the help of your healthcare provider, with the tools to improve your lifestyle and make active health decisions in how to live your life; it will help you live a healthy, active, and productive life.

Cervical cancer patients need to be monitored on a continuing basis often with Pap tests for a specified time frame by their gynecologist oncologist for disease recurrence. Depending on your stage and grade of the tumor, this may be for several years. Included in the examination may be a Pap test, a radiological evaluation like a computed tomography scan, or even a positron emission testing scan. After several normal tests, the surgeon may feel that you are ready to transfer your care to the local or community gynecologist for routine surveillance.

Living with a history of cancer really means that you will never be the same person as you were before the time of the cancer diagnosis. For cervical cancer patients, survivorship medicine includes the optimizing of general heath maintenance to prevent the development of secondary cancers whenever possible, and promoting health and well-being with an emphasis on primary and preventative care. This medical plan will encompass the screening for other cancers and prevention of chronic medical illnesses.

Survivorship medicine

The medical practice aimed at addressing the physical needs, long-term health, and life changes that result following the diagnosis and treatment for cancer.

SURVIVORSHIP ISSUES AFTER CERVICAL CANCER

60. Now that I have had cervical cancer, what do I do?

Cervical cancer survivors begin their journey once they hear the words "you have cancer." Once you recover from the initial shock of the diagnosis, cancer care becomes focused on "what I need to do now to get through this." However, after the initial treatment, most cancer survivors begin to question what else they can do to help decrease their risk for other cancers. Many focus on general health maintenance regimes and seek out many healthcare provider specialists to begin intensive screening programs. Others, who want to feel empowered and help maintain good health while minimizing their chances for recurrence, focus on optimum medical health and developing a wellness program/survivorship plan.

Cervical cancer survivors begin their journey once they hear the words "you have cancer."

As you move further away from your cancer treatment, you may find it difficult to adapt to life again. You are encouraged that your disease is stabilized or in remission; however, as a survivor, you want to optimize your health and prevent disease recurrence. Often there is lack of a social network or resources available to help you adjust to cancer survivorship.

61. How are women followed after treatment for cervical cancer?

According to the American College of Obstetricians and Gynecologists' technical bulletin on primary and preventative care on periodic assessment for women, some of the important components on a comprehensive physical examination include:

- Physical examination
    - Cardiac health (blood pressure, cholesterol screening)
    - Pelvic examination (Pap test)
    - Dental examinations and X-rays
    - Vision examinations
    - Diabetes screening with glucose checks

- Medication review of prescribed and over-the-counter medications, herbs and supplements (including vitamins), and prescription medications

- Tobacco, alcohol, and drug use screening

- Breast health and review of breast self-examination (mammography)

- Vaccinations

- Skin screening, sun health and skin cancer prevention

- Sexuality screening
    - Contraception
    - Reviewing safer sex practices and condom use
    - HIV and other sexually transmitted disease screening
    - Discussing how to prevent sexually transmitted diseases

- Nutrition and fitness
    - Evaluating diet and quantity of food and nutrition
    - Reinforcing portion size and food groups
    - Discussing alcohol and other substances
    - Reviewing exercise plan and time spent exercising

- Psychosocial evaluation

  Screening for psychiatric illnesses like depression and anxiety

  Evaluating employment satisfaction and enjoyment

  Ruling out job burnout and stress

  Screening for domestic partner abuse (physical, emotional, and sexual)

  Abuse history (sexual, physical, verbal, and emotional)

- Injury prevention

  Driving record and safety

  Safety belts

  Recreational hazards

  Firearms and storage issues

Perhaps one of the best references for general health maintenance for women is the American College of Obstetricians and Gynecologists' patient educational pamphlet published in 2007 entitled *Staying Healthy at All Ages*. This excellent booklet discusses screening, immunizations, and special needs as well as health tips for women of all ages. It can be obtained by contacting your obstetrician, gynecologist, or calling the American College directly. Speak with your doctor today about formulating a healthy plan to detect disease early, prevent other cancers, and stay healthy.

Your annual health examination is an important aspect of your overall health maintenance.

62. What should I know about my general health maintenance?

Your annual health examination is an important aspect of your overall health maintenance. A Pap test and cervical cancer screening should occur yearly or even twice a year depending on your cancer and how far you out are from your cancer treatment. Be certain to visit your gynecologist or internist on a regular basis. Pelvic and breast examinations also are very important components as well as discussions concerning smoking cessation and alcohol use. You may qualify for an annual mammogram and should be certain to perform breast self-examinations and report any abnormality to your doctor. Bone health and osteoporosis screening also are very important. Colonic health and prevention of colon cancer should be addressed.

If you are still having your menstrual cycles, contraception or birth control should be reviewed. Safe sex education, sexually transmitted infection protection, and the proper use of latex condoms and lubricants should be reviewed. Some tests that may be done are blood pressure measurements, height and weight, and other vital signs.

Monitoring your height and weight can be helpful with balancing nutrition and exercise regimes; obesity is a serious medical problem in U.S. society, and it is important to maintain a healthy weight. Periodically, you should also have your cholesterol and lipid profiles checked. Lipid profiles should be done every 5 years starting when you reach age 45. A thyroid-stimulating hormone test should be done annually starting at age 50, and you should have an annual immunization for influenza. It is also important to get a skin screening examination to have all your moles examined; skin cancer when caught early can be treated at a curable stage. In addition, it's very important to use sunscreens liberally when you are outside.

Some women may qualify for certain specific cancer screening programs like ovarian cancer screening,

SURVIVORSHIP ISSUES AFTER CERVICAL CANCER

depending on their family history. This specialized screening test consists of a transvaginal ultrasound to look at the ovaries as well as a blood test to measure CA125. Not all women qualify for these tests. You should consult with your healthcare provider to see if you are at an increased risk for ovarian cancer and would qualify for these tests, which can be incorporated into your annual visit to your healthcare provider.

Each woman's experience in survivorship is different. Allow yourself the luxury of feeling the way you feel; allow yourself the time to adapt to the cancer experience and incorporate it into your way of thinking.

As noted in another book in this series, ***100 Questions and Answers for Women Living with Cancer,*** women react differently on a psychological level to cancer; some women embrace survivorship, while others embark on a route of positive thinking and begin tai chi, yoga, meditation, and macrobiotic diets. Some women believe that bringing holistic mental treatments into the forefront of their survivorship experience is paramount when others focus primarily on getting back to their normal routine and work schedules. Each woman's experience in survivorship is different. Allow yourself the luxury of feeling the way you feel; allow yourself the time to adapt to the cancer experience and incorporate it into your way of thinking.

Reflexology

A complementary medicine practice that uses massage, squeezing, or pushing (normally of the feet or hands) to encourage positive effects on other body parts or provide a general sense of well-being.

Sometimes it does take a while to incorporate the experience into your way of life, but gradually you will face each new day with hope and excitement for your future. Unfortunately, some women face survivorship with concern, anxiety, and constant fear; fear of recurrence and an overwhelming fear of the cancer's return can be debilitating. The anniversary of the date of diagnosis or when their treatment was completed may be times when stress anxiety or low moods prevail. However, survivorship can bring feelings of new hope, happiness, and even excitement.

63. What are some techniques that can help me cope with cervical cancer?

Many different types of alternative therapies have been helpful when used by cancer patients; some can help keep stress to a minimum and relieve daily anxiety and pressures. Try one or another for a few weeks and see how you feel; if it works, keep with it; if not, then try another type. **Reflexology** is a practice that uses the application of pressure in different areas of the foot to relieve stress and pain. Massage like Shiatsu massage can involve gentle pressure and slow body stretching; a Swedish massage relieves tension by deeply kneading muscles. **Aromatherapy** uses inhaling specific scents (aromas) to help maintain bodily health. Essential oils are concentrated aromas that can be inhaled to promote a quiet sense of peace. Lavender, rosemary, or chamomile essence can be purchased at the local store; a few drops in bath water can be especially soothing. The gentle touch therapy of **Reiki** can promote a sense of calmness and tranquility. It may help you to reduce anxiety and maintain an ordered sense of calmness.

Many women find **meditation** very helpful; it involves breathing regulation and mind power. Using specific sitting postures and hand positions, you can gain inner calmness and serenity. **Yoga** is another popular exercise that many women use to help tone their bodies and relax their minds. Yoga consists of performing a series of stretching exercises and holding different postures while deeply breathing.

Other women find music very enjoyable, either playing an instrument or listening to their favorite composer. In **music therapy**, a woman listens to or plays a musical instrument in the company of a music therapist.

SURVIVORSHIP ISSUES AFTER CERVICAL CANCER

Aromatherapy
An integrative care practice that uses oils from plants to treat physical or psychological conditions. These oils are either inhaled or used in massage.

Reiki
A spiritual practice that uses healing energy to improve symptoms or treat conditions.

Meditation
A complementary medicine practice of concentrated attention toward a single point of reference.

Yoga
The spiritual practice aiming to unite the consciousness with universal consciousness to achieve harmony.

Music therapy
A complementary therapy practice using music to help psychologic or emotional adjustment before, during, or after cancer is diagnosed.

Depression is not seen as a sign of weakness; it is a known accepted biologic and medical illness that can be treated effectively with both medications and psychotherapy.

Sometimes you will feel sad. These feelings can persist for an extended period of time and are combined with feelings of depression, helplessness, or hopelessness. You can experience a loss of or an increased appetite, have sleep problems, and may suffer from depression or low moods that may warrant treatment by a psychiatrist. Depression is not seen as a sign of weakness; it is a known accepted biologic and medical illness that can be treated effectively with both medications and psychotherapy. The successful management of depression or severely low mood that interferes with activities of daily living can use one of many different types of antidepressant medications combined with psychotherapy. Many national cancer centers have posttreatment resource centers and survivorship programs that organize group support programs for female cancer survivors, and they are cancer diagnosis-specific. Share your specific concerns with your healthcare provider; he or she may be able to direct you to professional organizations or other healthcare providers that can help you regain your mental health. It is not something you should be ashamed about; many survivors face the same problems that you are going through, and emotional health is an important facet of your recovery.

64. I no longer have periods and my menopausal hot flashes are very troublesome. What can I do?

Chemical menopause

Induction of menopause by the use of treatments that are toxic to the ovaries; includes such treatments as radiation, chemotherapy, or hormonal.

Surgical menopause

The complete stop of a woman's periods that occurs as a result of the removal of the ovaries.

Many cervical cancer patients go through abrupt menopause or when a woman does not have a menstrual cycle for 1 year. **Chemical menopause** occurs when the woman has received chemicals (like chemotherapy) or medications that temporarily or permanently stop her cycles. **Surgical menopause** occurs when both ovaries are removed so hormones are no longer produced. There is a grouping of symptoms that often accompany menopause, and the most troublesome include hot flashes and vaginal dryness.

The exact reason and cause for hot flashes is not yet known. However, some researchers think that a hormone called **luteinizing hormone (LH)** is released at the same time as the levels of estrogen decrease. This release of LH may effect a change in veins getting larger, which may cause skin flushing, increased sweating with increased blood flow, increased body temperature, and a rapid heart rate. Some women feel as if they are perspiring, soaking through their clothing.

Hot flashes can begin as a sensation of pressure or warm heat in the head, neck, chest, and back, which spreads to the entire body. They can begin several years before menses stops completely in the **perimenopausal** period (transition years). Hot flashes can interfere with a good night's rest, which may make you irritable and anxious the following morning.

Each woman's experience with hot flashes is of course unique, and many women experience hot flashes that are not bothersome and do not warrant therapy. Others are debilitated and cannot function on a day-to-day basis because of their severe menopausal syndrome. Quality-of-life issues are paramount, and each woman must decide for herself if her hot flashes need therapy. There are many different methods to treat hot flashes, and each woman should decide what is best and safest for her. It is always best to consult with your healthcare team about your symptoms and which treatment option is best for you specifically.

Luteinizing hormone (LH)
A hormone produced by the pituitary gland that is necessary for reproductive function. Rises in LH trigger an egg to be released from the ovary.

Perimenopausal
The time in which women are having irregular periods, right before the periods completely stop.

SURVIVORSHIP ISSUES AFTER CERVICAL CANCER

91

Progesterone

A hormone in women that is required for normal periods, maintaining pregnancy, and the development of the fetus.

Hormone therapy (HT)

The use of medications to modify or replace the hormones a body makes or lacks. In the case of cancer, hormone therapy may be those medications that block hormones from feeding a cancer cell. However, in the case of hot flashes, it may denote medications given to enhance low levels of hormones that result from menopause.

65. What are the most accepted treatment methods for hot flashes?

Hormonal therapy with estrogen and **progesterone** is the mainstay treatment for hot flashes. However in recent years, **hormone therapy (HT)** has gotten a lot of negative publicity press since the recent publication of the Women's Health Initiative study, which publicized the possible association of estrogen and progesterone replacement with a slightly increased risk for heart attacks, breast cancer, and strokes. Practically overnight, many women stopped taking their hormonal pills and safety concerns were heralded as the reasoning to stop taking theses pills. According to the American Medical Association, only about 7.6 million women used hormones in 2004 when in 2002 there were close to 18.5 million users.

Despite these findings, HT of estrogen alone or in combination with progesterone still remains an effective treatment for troublesome hot flashes. There are many new and effective low-dose preparations that come in all forms of delivery systems, including a patch that is placed on your skin in differing areas, rings that can be placed within the vagina, gels (can be applied to the body), vaginal tablets, creams, and other formulations. The North American Menopause Society advocates that only severe and debilitating hot flashes are to be treated and if hormones are to be used, one should be using the lowest doses for the shortest amount of time for hot flash and other symptom relief. If you still have a uterus, progesterone should be added to your hormonal regime to prevent endometrial thickening or hyperplasia.

Every woman should carefully educate herself and analyze the risks and benefit of taking hormones, especially with regards to her symptoms and family and personal history. It is important to discuss your concerns regarding hormones with your doctor.

If you do decide to take hormones, continue to have your physical examinations, clinical breast examination, and annual mammogram. Breast self-examinations and a risk assessment also should be done on a regular basis. If any of your close family members including sisters, mothers, aunts, or other close relatives develop cancers, discuss your continuation of the hormones with your doctor. It is important to report any side effects like abnormal vaginal bleeding to your doctor.

Recently, reports in the media have advocated compounded **bioidentical hormones** as a safe alternative to hormone replacement therapy. These are plant-derived hormones that are created, mixed, and packaged by a pharmacist who can customize the product according to the physician's specifications. However, according to the American College of Obstetricians and Gynecologists, most compounded products have not undergone strict scientific study and there may be concerns about the safety, purity, and efficacy of these products; for this reason, bioidentical hormones are not safer than those prescribed by your doctor. If you are considering taking bioidentical hormones or are now taking a prescribed compound, it may be dangerous for your continued health. It is strongly recommended that you discuss the risks of bioidentical hormones with your cancer specialist and gynecologist.

Bioidentical hormones

Hormonal preparations, usually animal or plant derived, that have a similar chemical structure to a human's naturally occurring hormones.

66. I don't want to take hormones. What else can I do to manage my hot flashes?

Even though it may be safe for most cervical cancer patients to use estrogen alone or a combination of estrogen and progesterone therapies, many women choose not to use these products because of personal choice or fear of developing breast cancer or another type of hormonally sensitive cancer. There are a variety of methods to decrease the severity and intensity of hot flashes. Some include environmental changes like wearing absorbent, cotton clothing or dressing in layers so that the outermost layers can be removed when you get a hot flash. In addition, there is specialty designer sleepwear that has been developed for those with night-time hot flashes and sweats. Drinking an ice-cold glass of water, putting a cold moist compress on your face, or using a misting-type bottle can help you feel cooler in the middle of a flash. Try to lower your thermostat and place a room fan near where you sleep. Hand-held fans also can be helpful. Some women find biofeedback techniques and relaxation techniques like yoga, medi-tation, and tai chi to be helpful for troublesome hot flashes. Regular exercise, avoiding cigarette smoking, and hot baths also can be helpful. Some women try to do paced respirations to help the intensity of hot flashes. Sometimes changes in diet can help with hot flashes; it may mean avoiding certain triggers like caf-feine, alcohol (including beer, wine, and liquor), and spicy foods. Consider adding some vitamin supple-ments such as vitamin B_6 (200 or 250 mg daily) or Peridin C (two tablets three times a day). Start with these over-the-counter medicines and allow at least 4 to 6 weeks for them to work. If possible, add one supple-ment at a time so that you can determine if it's work-ing for you.

Drinking an ice-cold glass of water, putting a cold moist compress on your face, or using a misting-type bottle can help you feel cooler in the middle of a flash.

Acupuncture is the ancient Chinese medical system where very thin needles are painlessly and strategically placed into the skin. It is used to help control chronic pain in addition to healing a wide variety of other ail-

Acupuncture

A traditional Chinese practice of treating a health condition or medical state by inserting needles into the skin at specific points to unblock the flow of energy.

ments. Acupuncture works by stimulating specific portions of the nervous system, relieving pain by causing signal transmitters and hormones in the brain to work in different ways. Many women report relief from hot flashes with acupuncture.

Sometimes, prescription medications such as antihypertensive medications (clonidine and methyl dopa) and antidepressants (like selective serotonin reuptake inhibitors) can be prescribed to help minimize hot flashes. Antiepileptic medications like gabapentin also may be effective pharmacological therapy for the hot-flash sufferer; however, they do have some common side effects. It is always important to talk with your doctor or nurse about your medications to see if you should try another type of medicine and discuss possible side effects. Remember that all medications have some side effects so, in addition to discussing this with your clinician, it is best to carefully read the package insert that comes with the prescription.

67. My vagina is so dry. How can I keep my vagina tissue healthy?

With the treatment of cervical cancer, you may have gone into premature menopause where your hormonal levels decrease. The vaginal tissues naturally become dry as a woman's estrogen levels decrease. This sometimes leads to troublesome symptoms of itchiness, burning, irritation, and painful intercourse. Luckily, there are many methods to treat the symptoms of vaginal dryness or vaginal atrophy.

When a woman ages, the vagina naturally becomes dry and less elastic. Cancer treatments can worsen these changes, and it is not uncommon for cervical cancer survivors to complain of dryness in the vaginal area. Some women take estrogen either by a pill, patch, cream, ring, or gel to prevent anatomical changes; some, however, may be concerned about estrogen and its theoretical links to cancers like breast cancer.

Vaginal moisturizers and lubricants may be helpful in maintaining vaginal health, especially for women who want to begin with less-aggressive methods to maintain vaginal health. A vitamin E capsule can be punctured with a pin and then inserted into your vagina. Another method is to empty the capsule's gel content onto your finger and insert vaginally. Replens is a vaginal moisturizer that can be purchased over the counter and comes with an easily filled applicator. You can use either moisturizer two to three times a week. Be sure to read the ingredients of the moisturizers because many can contain bactericides, spermicidal components, colors, flavors, and other additives that can be irritating to the vagina. Vaginal moisturizers should be used on a regular basis because they help hydrate the vaginal lining and help restore vaginal elasticity and stretchability.

Vaginal lubricants are typically used to make sexual intercourse more pleasurable. There are many common types that can be purchased at the pharmacy or grocery store. A good lubricant should be water based and compatible with rubber products like condoms. Menopausal women should avoid all petroleum-based products such as mineral oil, petroleum jelly, and edible oils or other liquid food products. These often upset the delicate balance between the good and bad bacteria within the vagina and result in vaginal infections; they also can affect the utility of condoms.

Local vaginal hormones that come in creams, gels rings, and tablets are the most common types of minimally absorbed vaginal estrogen products that provide small doses of estrogen directly in the vagina. Vaginal and vulvar creams typically are applied to both the interior of the vagina and exterior of the **vaginal vault**. The estradiol vaginal ring can be placed within the vaginal vault for 3 months before it needs to be replaced. Minimally absorbed 17-beta estradiol vaginal tablets are another type of vaginal hormone replacement. These tablets are contained in a plastic disposable applicator that can be inserted into your vagina every night for 14 days, and then twice a week, at bedtime. The long-term safety for all minimally absorbed vaginal estrogen products needs to be further studied, especially in larger populations.

Ask your doctor, nurse practitioner, or other healthcare providers about which type of treatment is best for you given your cancer, stage, and treatment. Perhaps local estrogen is appropriate for you and it would be helpful.

68. Should I be worried about my bone health?

Osteoporosis is a significant medical illness that affects both men and women as they age. Bone loss can lead to chronic back pain, pain when you are walking, deformity of the bones or spine, and if your treatment for cervical cancer has caused premature menopause or removal of the ovaries, you may be at risk for bone loss and osteoporosis.

With the loss of hormones (especially estrogens) and with the natural process of aging, your bones can lose their density, and become thin, weak, and fragile. There are a number of risks associated with lowered bone-mass density, and they include a previous fracture, being a woman, age (older women are at a greater risk), and

Vaginal vault
The area at the top of the vagina, adjacent to the cervix.

Osteoporosis
Bony degeneration; also known as osteoarthritis.

SURVIVORSHIP ISSUES AFTER CERVICAL CANCER

family history (you are at a greater risk for osteoporosis if your mother or grandmother had osteoporosis). Some chronic medical conditions like rheumatoid arthritis, thyroid dysfunction, kidney and liver disease as well as some gastrointestinal disorders, a sedentary (nonactive) lifestyle, smoking, and excessive alcohol consumption and medications like steroids, thyroid replacement, blood thinners, or antiseizure medications also are considered risk factors. Bone-density testing involves a dual energy X-ray absorptionmetry scan or bone densitometry. These are painless tests that assess the bone quality in a variety of bodily locations like the spine, the leg, and sometimes the wrist and ankle bones. Most insurance will pay for the test every 2 years after the time when women have gone into natural or surgically or chemically induced menopause. Calcium and exercise typically have been the mainstays for bone preservation. A calcium supplement may help you to maintain bone strength. It is always best to consult with your healthcare provider to discuss how much (**dosage**) and how often you should be taking calcium because the body can absorb only a certain amount of calcium at a time. Because many women already are taking a multivitamin that contains a calcium supplement, it is best to discuss calcium with your healthcare provider. Calcium has the potential to interfere with other medications you may be taking. There are ongoing and heated debates about the usefulness of calcium supplementation. Controversy appears both in the medical journals and the media. Researchers now are questioning whether calcium supplementation is actually beneficial to overall bone health and maintenance. How much of the calcium do you actually need? How much does the body absorb? Does calcium really impact bone health? Until

Dosage

The amount or volume to be taken, as generally prescribed by a healthcare provider.

the final solution is decided, one should eat a well-balanced diet that is rich in a variety of healthy foods that contain calcium; discuss supplementation with your doctor.

If increased exercise and calcium intake do not maintain (stabilize) your bone loss, your healthcare provider may suggest a medication in the class called **bisphosphonates**. The most commonly prescribed medications are risedronate and alendronate. Both these medications need to be taken on an empty stomach, with the person sitting upright for at least one half hour; the dose can be on a once-a-week schedule. The most common side effects are upper gastrointestinal upset and irritation. A newer medication on the market is ibandronate sodium, which is a tablet taken once a month.

Still, these drugs are not without their own side effects. One of the more widely publicized medical concerns involves the development of jaw **osteonecrosis**. This is an extremely rare occurrence that has been reported in some patients receiving biphosphonates. Osteonecrosis occurs when the blood supply to the bone is interrupted (temporarily or permanently), which causes the bone tissue to die and—if untreated—the bone may collapse.

Exercise, especially weight-bearing activities like walking, jogging, walking up stairs, or climbing, has been proven to maintain bone health and overall excellent health. Even activities like dancing and weight training can help with bone preservation. Make a conscious decision to join the gym, begin walking after work, or just enjoy a nice day in the park strolling around. Exercise is important for overall health, fitness, and well-being.

Biphosphonate
A class of drugs that are used to prevent or treat osteoporosis or bone degeneration.

Osteonecrosis
The process describing bone death.

SURVIVORSHIP ISSUES AFTER CERVICAL CANCER

99

69. I would like to prevent other cancers. What can I do?

Different organizations and various task forces periodically publish patient care guidelines about how people should be screened for a specific disease. For example, the American Cancer Society, American College of Obstetricians and Gynecologists, and other associations like the U.S. Preventative Services Task Force, American College of Cardiology, and American Association of Gastrointestinal Surgeons all produce various age-specific guidelines as to when women should get periodically screened. Because many of these guidelines are conflicting and you can become confused, it is best to formulate a healthcare plan with your trusted healthcare team. Different women are at risk for differing cancers, so it is best to individualize your plan.

The bottom line is that your care needs to be tailored to your specific history and your specific medical needs. You will definitely need Pap test screening of the **vaginal cuff** even if your cervix, uterus, and ovaries have been removed. Typically your gynecologist oncologist will perform these for several years after your cancer treatment to ensure that you have not had a cancer recurrence.

If you still have your uterus—and because there is no screening test for uterine cancer—women who experience any type of abnormal vaginal bleeding and who are at risk should consult their healthcare provider immediately. They may need an appropriate evaluation that could include an **endometrial biopsy** and a **transvaginal ultrasound**.

The **vulva** is considered the outer part of the female reproductive tract and sometimes is called the lips of the

Your care needs to be tailored to your specific history and your specific medical needs.

Vaginal cuff

The part created by a surgeon at the top of the vagina following removal of the cervix.

Endometrial biopsy

The process of obtaining tissue from the uterine lining.

Transvaginal ultrasound

A radiology test in which the probe (on the ultrasound) is inserted directly into the vagina. It is the most accurate way to evaluate a woman's reproductive organs.

Vulva

The external female genitals that are seen when a woman is naked.

pelvis. Cancer of the vulva and **clitoris** are rather rare, and early diagnosis and treatments are needed to prevent extensive spread of the disease. Smoking, HPV infection, multiple sexual partners, HIV infection, or a history of cervical abnormalities all may contribute to the development of vulvar cancer. Because there is no recommended screening test to detect vulvar or clitoral cancer, it is important to note if you have any unusual symptoms including itchiness, burning in the vulvar area, dry scaly skin changes or bleeding, or abnormal discharge from the vulvar area. You should report these changes to your doctor, and you may need a small outpatient biopsy to get a definitive diagnosis of the troubling area. Many women perform self vulvar examination with the aid of a hand-held mirror and report any changes in skin color or changes in surface texture to the doctor.

Ovarian cancer does not have any specific, clear-cut presenting symptoms. Very often, patients present with disease that is advanced in stage and has spread to many pelvic or abdominal organs. Some of the vague symptoms associated with ovarian cancer may be abdominal gas or unexplained bloating that does not go away, pelvic pressure, or a swollen abdomen. Recent research indicates that some women complain of urinary symptoms in the early stages of ovarian cancer. If you are at an increased risk because of your ethnicity, genetic problems, a strong family history for either breast or ovarian cancer, or a personal history of breast cancer before the age of 50, you may be eligible for ovarian cancer screening. Presently screening includes a transvaginal ultrasound to assess the ovaries, regular pelvic examinations, and blood testing to measure CA125 (cancer antigen 125, which measures a sugar protein that increases when tissues are inflamed or damaged).

Clitoris
A woman's highly sensitive pelvic organ that is associated with orgasm.

SURVIVORSHIP ISSUES AFTER CERVICAL CANCER

101

Many cancer institutions have functionalized screening programs so you can have a regular visit scheduled every 6 months with your healthcare provider. Screening is recommended only for those at higher risk for developing ovarian cancer. The test is not 100 percent specific and sensitive, which means that while the test may show abnormalities, it does not mean that you have cancer. Ovarian cancer screening testing may cause a lot of anxiety for the patient because very often the scan finds harmless simple pelvic cysts that require close follow-up and extensive evaluations.

Many women of all races, socioeconomic backgrounds, religions, and social standing will develop breast cancer over the course of their lifetime, and one in seven women will develop breast cancer in her lifetime. Breast health awareness is important so that you can maintain excellent breast health. Some of the myths concerning breast cancer should be dispelled. At the present time, there are no accurate scientific data that directly link underwire bras, antiperspirant usage, or having had an elective termination of pregnancy with breast cancer.

Mammography (a special X-ray of the breast where the radiation exposure of the breast tissue is minimal), clinical breast examination by a physician, and breast self-examination are three of the best techniques to help detect breast disease at an early stage.

Mammography (a special X-ray of the breast where the radiation exposure of the breast tissue is minimal), clinical breast examination by a physician, and breast self-examination are three of the best techniques to help detect breast disease at an early stage. All three contribute to excellent breast health. The American Cancer Society recommends that women get annual mammograms beginning at the age of 40. After that mammograms should be repeated every 1 to 2 years until the age of 50, when they should be done on an annual basis. The screening program should be individualized according to risk factors and family history. Breast self-examination for women over the age of 20 is advocated on a monthly basis, and clinical breast examination by a healthcare professional should be a part of the routine annual health maintenance examination. On the day of your mammogram, you should not use deodorant or antiperspirant, because some contain certain ingredients that can interfere with correct interpretation of the mammogram. Wear a two-piece outfit, because you will need to be undressed from the waist up for the mammogram procedure. The best time to have a mammogram is shortly after your menstrual cycle. Always follow up and call your gynecologist or healthcare provider if you do not receive your mammogram results within a few days after the test.

According to the Cancer Research and Prevention Foundation, colon cancer is the second leading cause of cancer deaths in the United States. Close to 145,000 women and men are diagnosed, and between 55,000 and 56,000 die each year from the disease. When discovered early, colon cancer is treatable and often curable. Colon cancer is a serious medical illness for women, and most medical associations advocate colon screening starting at the age of 50. There are several methods to screen for colon cancer. Some include a **fecal occult blood test** for which you will be given a home testing card kit. You are asked to get a sample of stool on the card, insert it into the supplied plastic sleeve, and mail it to a laboratory. The card sample then is tested for the presence or absence of blood. Other tests are a flexible sigmoidoscopy (every 5 years), colonoscopy, and double-contrast barium enema. It is understandable that you may be fearful or embarrassed about the colon, but you must remember that rectal screening is one of the positive steps you can take toward disease discovery and early effective treatment. A **colonoscopy** is a medical outpatient surgical procedure

Mammography

A special X-ray of the breast that is used as a screening tool for breast cancer.

SURVIVORSHIP ISSUES AFTER CERVICAL CANCER

Fecal occult blood test

A noninvasive test that checks for blood in the stool.

Colonoscopy

A diagnostic test for evaluating the colon.

that is the screening tool to detect colonic abnormalities and precancerous growths in the colon. It looks at the large intestine or colon and rectum. It is the best type of test that can image the lining (colonic mucosa) and can be used to accurately identify colon cancer. After a special preparation that cleanses the colon, a small tube, which is thin and flexible and has a small video camera with a light source at the end, is placed within the rectum and advanced so that the gastrointestinal specialist can see the entire lining of the colon. The tube is lubricated so that it can be advanced into the colon with little discomfort. You will have received some sedation before the procedure, so you will be in a relaxed state of mind called "**twilight.**" You will be conscious but unable to recall all of the details of the procedure.

Sun health is very important to prevent damage from the sun and skin cancer. Limit your exposure to the sun during the times when the sun is the most harmful, from 10 AM to 4 PM; cover the parts of your body exposed to the sun with long-sleeved, lightweight clothing. Seek shade and wear hats that shield your face, ears, head, and neck, and wear eye protection against the sun's damaging rays. The liberal use of a nonexpired sunscreen that has a minimum sun protection factor of 15 and that can block both the UVA and UVB rays of the sun is essential. You should apply a sunscreen often and liberally, whether on sunny or cloudy/hazy days. Sunscreens should be applied approximately 30 minutes before exposure to the sun and should be applied repeatedly, especially when engaging in water sports, swimming, or other activities that have caused a lot of perspiration.

Twilight

A state induced with medication that allows sedation, making invasive procedures more comfortable. Ideally, medications will induce a state of sleep in which the person closes the eyes and rests while the procedure is performed.

70. Should I stop smoking? What about alcohol?

Health problems associated with smoking are well known. There is a strong association of a variety of cancers with tobacco use. Lung, throat, and tongue cancers all are associated with tobacco smoking. Smoke also has been associated with kidney, bladder, voice box (larynx), and cervical cancer, and even some types of leukemia. Cigarette smoking contributes to a variety of medical illnesses, including emphysema, bronchitis, peripheral vascular disease, and cardiac illness. Most cancer institutions, including the American Cancer Association, have formalized smoking cessation programs that can help you stop smoking if you have not done so already. Some of the nicotine replacement options are a patch, inhaler, chewing gum, or spray. The side effects of nicotine replacement therapy include headaches, dizziness, stomach upset, visual changes, unusual dreams or nightmares, or diarrhea. The medication Bupropion can be used to help someone quit smoking. Although it is classified as an antidepressant medication, it can be used in combination with nicotine replacement therapy and a formalized smoking cessation program.

Although a moderate amount of alcohol consumption has been linked to a decrease in cardiovascular disease, drinking more than two alcoholic beverages per day is associated with increased risks for developing breast cancer and other diseases. According to the American Cancer Society, excessive alcohol consumption has been linked to a variety of cancers including cancer of the tongue, esophagus, pharynx, larynx, and liver. It is estimated that women who drink two to five alcoholic

According to the American Cancer Society, excessive alcohol consumption has been linked to a variety of cancers including cancer of the tongue, esophagus, pharynx, larynx, and liver.

105

beverages daily have a one and a half times higher risk of developing breast malignancy. Some key concepts to remember are that one alcoholic beverage is defined as a regular 12-ounce beer, a 5-ounce glass of white or red wine, or 1.5 ounces of 80 proof (percent) hard liquor (such as scotch, bourbon, gin, or vodka). Women who are pregnant, small young children, and young adults who are not of legal drinking age should never consume alcohol. Alcohol interferes with many prescription medications and impacts your ability to react quickly. It is always best to avoid driving an automobile or operating dangerous equipment after alcohol consumption. Moderation is the rule with alcohol consumption.

PART ELEVEN

Sexuality After Cervical Cancer

Is it safe to have sex after
treatment for cervical cancer?

Do many cervical cancer survivors
experience sexual complaints?

What are the causes of sexual problems
in the cervical cancer survivor?

More . . .

71. Is it safe to have sex after treatment for cervical cancer?

Sexual concerns are common and many cancer survivors face the additional issues of a changed self-image, fatigue from their cancer therapies, and mortality. Although not life threatening, not having a healthy and active sex life can affect your entire relationship with your spouse or partner as well as how you feel about yourself. The ramifications from cancer and its treatment can have a serious affect on your sexual satisfaction, and the complaint is extremely prevalent in all women of all ages and for all cancer types. It is important to ask your healthcare professional for help!

Although not life threatening, not having a healthy and active sex life can affect your entire relationship with your spouse or partner as well as how you feel about yourself.

72. Do many cervical cancer survivors experience sexual complaints?

Some cervical cancer survivors complain of having a low **libido** (hypoactive desire disorder), changes in orgasm, or arousal. Sexual pain disorders like **dyspareunia** (pain during intercourse) and **vaginismus** (reflexive contracture of the pelvic and vaginal muscles) also are prevalent. Because surgery may shorten the vagina or radiation may damage the vaginal lining, it is important to discuss your concerns regarding sexual function with your healthcare team. A detailed assessment will include a completed medical and gynecological history, comprehensive general physical and genital examination, and a psychosexual examination. Laboratory blood tests of various hormones or radiological evaluation may be appropriate. Patients are encouraged to see a sexual medicine specialist/gynecologist.

Libido
A person's sex drive.

Dyspareunia
Pain with sexual intercourse.

Vaginismus
An involuntary tightening of the vaginal muscles when the vagina is penetrated. This action can cause significant pain.

109

Sexual dysfunction is often complex and multidimensional, so an individual's treatment regimen may involve several different approaches. Healthy, satisfying sexual functioning and treatment success are impacted by a variety of factors including medical illnesses, hormonal levels, relationship concerns, partner availability, underlying psychiatric disorders, general medical well-being, and cultural and religious behaviors. According to 2005 statistics from the American Cancer Society, with technological treatments and advancements in diagnostics and therapeutics, an estimated 60 percent of all cancer survivors will live at least 5 years after their diagnosis. Know that you are not alone if you have some sexual complaints. Don't feel embarrassed or ashamed about discussing the issues with your doctors. Once you have discussed your concerns, your physician should be receptive to helping you with these deeply private issues. Sexuality and intimacy are critical for health happiness and feeling connected with both yourself and your partner.

73. What are the causes of sexual problems in the cervical cancer survivor?

A variety of factors can interfere with a woman's sexuality. In addition to her psychological make-up and past experience with intimate relationships and medications, other cancer treatments may affect how a woman may respond sexually. Removal of the uterus, ovaries, cervix, and perhaps part of the vagina may affect your self-esteem and influence how you view yourself as a woman. With extensive surgical resection and radical surgery, women may mourn the loss of their youthful body and femininity. Large tumor resections that involve extensive physical changes, such as bowel removal, may result in functional changes such as ileostomies, colonostomies, and ileoconduits that may be perceived as embarrassing or ugly. Surgical scarring after procedures may interfere with extremity mobility, and even determining a comfortable sexual position may be challenging.

Radiation therapy may cause skin and vaginal changes like thickening, contractures, or cause different textures and decreased lubrication. Some other side effects from radiation can include fatigue, loss of hair on your head or in the genital area, diarrhea, nausea, and vomiting. All these issues may contribute to a lack of interest and lowered libido. Patients and/or their partners may have unfounded concerns regarding the myth of being "radioactive." Because some cervical cancer patients do have an implant, they are receiving localized radiation, once it is removed; the woman is no longer radioactive. The truth is that you cannot catch radiation nor are you considered radioactive if you have undergone radiation treatment.

The truth is that you cannot catch radiation nor are you considered radioactive if you have undergone radiation treatment.

Vaginal fibrosis with stiffening and hardening of a shortened vaginal vault can be caused by direct radiation to the vagina. This can seriously impact a woman's capacity for penetrative intercourse and affect her genital pelvic and perhaps her clitoral sensitivity. Her sexual sensation or orgasms may be less intense than before, so it may take longer to reach the same level of excitement and arousal. You may be instructed and encouraged to use **vaginal dilators** as part of your postoperative care plan to maintain vaginal length and integrity. Continued use of dilators with consistent follow-up with your sexual healthcare provider can help maintain the capacity for vaginal intercourse.

Vaginal fibrosis
The narrowing or scarring of the vagina. It can make sex extremely painful for women.

Vaginal dilators
Medical plastic applicators that help restore the vaginal muscles so that they are more adaptable.

SEXUALITY AFTER CERVICAL CANCER

Chemotherapy
Medications that cause cells to stop dividing; used in the treatment of cancer.

Chemotherapy can cause nausea, diarrhea, and membrane irritation and can induce premature menopause, which can present as hot flashes and vaginal dryness or atrophy. Loss of hair on the head, eyebrows, eyelashes, and genitals is distressing and affects a female's perception of sexual attractiveness. Chemotherapy-induced early ovarian failure causes menopausal symptoms like hot flashes, sleep problems, vaginal dryness, and mood problems. Vaginal dryness can become a serious medical concern and often leads to painful intercourse on penetration.

Darlene's comment:

I feel the causes are vaginal discomfort due to dryness and the narrowing of the vagina from radiation.

Many women report continued feelings of low moods, melancholy, or depressive symptoms about their body image, fear of cancer recurrence, and sexuality problems even after their successful cancer treatments.

74. What are the psychological changes after cancer that may impact sexual functioning?

Many women report continued feelings of low moods, melancholy, or depressive symptoms about their body image, fear of cancer recurrence, and sexuality problems even after their successful cancer treatments and they are deemed cancer free. Some women are upset about negative sexual experiences that happened in the past whether they involved episodes of promiscuity, extramarital affairs, and/or the experience of sexually transmitted diseases that may incorrectly transfer these experiences to their genital cancer diagnosis. Underlying preexisting psychiatric illnesses combined with depressed and lowered moods can affect sexual self-image, as well, and contribute to the development of female sexual complaints. Many women fear that they will no longer be attractive and no longer be able to attract a sexual partner. Words like "damaged" are often used by these women.

Relationship dynamics also can change once the woman has experienced a cervical cancer diagnosis. The healthy partner may have a family role reversal. He or she may become the caregiver and/or primary or solo wage earner, which may lead to difficult adjustments to their altered familial roles. Marital and financial tension can be stressful and cause a breakdown in communication for the couple. Other stressors include the threat of disease recurrence, early death and disability, and bodily disfigurement as well as economic pressures, work-related difficulties, and medical insurance costs and coverage.

It is important to understand your feelings after a cancer diagnosis. If this is impacting your ability to have meaningful relationships or is impacting your ability to maintain social connections, business obligations, or is interfering with your quality of life, then it is possible that you have a medical depression. If your feelings of isolation and sadness are overwhelming, then it is perfectly acceptable to seek medical and psychological counseling. Depression is a medical illness that requires treatment; do not be scared or fear that you will be judged for your low mood; it is common and many cancer survivors suffer from low mood changes.

Darlene's comment:

After my hysterectomy, I was so scared to have intercourse. I was afraid that it was going to be very painful.

75. What specific sexual health management therapies can I expect when I seek treatments as a female cancer survivor?

The treatment of female sexual complaints is complex and involves the combined approach of treating the woman's medicine issues as well as assessing and treating her sexual psychological issues. Listed here are a variety of therapeutic options that the sexual medicine specialist may perform to effectively treat your sexual complaints.

Cancer survivors often have other underlying medical conditions and illnesses that directly impact on their sexual health and the sexual response cycle. Evaluation and treatment of chronic illnesses, such as uncontrolled hypertension, hypercholesterolemia, and/or an underlying thyroid dysfunction, arthritis, or diabetes can be simple to identify. Diagnosis and treatment of underlying genital infections like candida (yeast), bacterial vaginosis, and *Trichomoniais* and screening bloodwork can rule out underlying chronic illnesses. Hormonal levels of estrogens, testosterones, and progesterone as well as other hormonal profiles typically are measured, too.

Most classes of drugs can affect the female sexual response cycle and cause sexual problems. Many antidepressants, antihypertensive medications, and oral contraceptives can change sexual desire, arousal, and orgasm. Ask your physicians to check pharmacologic guides to identify potential offending agents and consider substituting another drug. Patients with sexual complaints are always encouraged to make lifestyle modifications that will enhance and improve their quality of life. A well-balanced nutritious diet, an active aerobic exercise plan, stopping the use of tobacco and illicit drugs, and minimizing alcohol consumption are encouraged. Some specific sexually structured tasks and behavior modification techniques include erotic reading, sensate focusing, squeeze-stop technique, guided imagery, exploration of sexual fantasies, and masturbation exercises.

Patients and their partners may be encouraged to engage in alternative sexual positions. Most couples engage in intercourse in the missionary position, which may facilitate deep penetration. This position, however, can be very painful for the woman who has a shortened vagina as a result of surgery and or radiation from cervical cancer treatment. Try alternative positions like side-to-side (spooning) or a female superior position, which may help limit deep pelvic thrusting and minimize vaginal discomfort during intercourse.

If pain is a concern, try sexual intimacy when pain is at low level with minimal fatigue. Techniques such as warm soaks and physical therapy help loosen tense muscles. Guided imagery, meditation, deep-muscle relaxation, and avoidance of exhaustion are options that should be explored. Specifically trained pain management specialists can be consulted to adjust or reduce opioid regimens and add adjunctive or alternative analgesics to lessen fatigue while maintaining sufficient pain relief.

There is a wide variety of take-home items, such as pamphlets, books, videos, and other visual aids, which provide educational reinforcement and serve as a future reference. You may opt to search the Internet when seeking information concerning the treatment of your sexual problems. The Women's Sexual Health Foundation, the International Society for the Study of Women's Sexual Health, North American Menopause Society, and the American College of Obstetricians and Gynecologists are all organizations that maintain wonderful information on their Web sites concerning sexual health and sexual education. They also provide medical information about the latest updates on female sexual therapeutics. For the female cancer survivor, the American Cancer Society's booklet entitled *Cancer and Sexuality* is an excellent patient reference guide. It provides factual information and helpful suggestions to maintain and improve your sexual functioning.

Because women's sexual complaints are a complex phenomenon and situational issues are a fundamental part of the diagnosis, a comprehensive treatment regime would not be complete without appropriate sexual counseling and therapy. Sexual complaints are best treated by a certified sexual therapist who is educated and trained to deal with patients with sexual complaints. Psychotherapists, psychologists, and physical therapists can be extremely effective when vaginal dilators are prescribed for the treatment of vaginismus, during which a woman's muscles in her vagina close tightly, almost involuntarily.

Local and national support organizations like the American Association for Sex Education, Counseling and Treatment (http://www.aasect.org) and the Association of Reproductive Health Professionals can provide further information and support to help patients achieve greater comfort with these issues, both within their relationships and families and within themselves.

76. What pharmacologic interventions can improve my sexual function?

Systemic and local estrogen replacement remains the mainstay in the management of female sexual dysfunction. Estrogen is one of many important hormones that are necessary for many aspects of sexual function in women. Central arousal and peripheral and pelvic sexual response are dependent on estrogen levels and in some instances testosterone levels as well. Systemic hormonal replacement can be achieved with a variety of products either taken orally or transdermally (through a skin patch).

Estrogen is one of many important hormones that are necessary for many aspects of sexual function in women.

For women who have an intact uterus and did not undergo a hysterectomy, the standard of care is to add a progesterone hormone to the regime; this prevents endometrial overgrowth and endometrial cancer. Newer low dosages of hormone replacement are now available. With the emerging data from the Woman's Health Initiative study, there are growing concerns about both estrogen and progesterone hormones and potential associated risks of cardiovascular events or breast cancer. Risks and benefit profiles should be discussed with your healthcare and sexual medicine specialist.

Estrogen has many effects on the genital system. It promotes cell maturation and proliferation and increases blood flow, but also stimulates secretions. A decrease of estrogen causes decreased blood supply to the genitals, increased dryness, and can lead to painful intercourse and possibly a reactive lowered desire. The use of local vaginal estrogen (creams, rings, and tablets) for the treatment of vaginal atrophy is available and widely accepted. Many products are minimally absorbed such as estrogen vaginal tablets or estrogen rings. Cream preparations can provide relief from irritation of the pelvic areas, including the vagina and vulva.

Some sexual health providers prefer to prescribe a minimally absorbed local 17β-estradiol tablet, which is minimally absorbed into the systemic circulation. It is important to recognize that estrogen use is not without risks or complications. Some of the side effects include possible blood clots (thromboembolic events), increased heart problems (cardiovascular events), an increase in breast cancer, and increased endometrial cancer if unopposed with a progestin. Talk with your clinician to analyze which one may be the right solution for you and your partner.

77. What is testosterone replacement and how is it linked with women's sexuality?

Testosterone

A sexual hormone produced in the ovaries that is important in normal sexual functioning.

Female androgen insufficiency syndrome

A constellation of symptoms attributed to low testosterone levels in women including unexplained fatigue, decreased well-being, lack of energy or motivation, and decreased sexual function.

Replacement of **testosterone** in females remains controversial, and many researchers are still unconvinced about any direct linkage between testosterone and female sexual health. **Female androgen insufficiency syndrome** is a medical condition characterized by decreased motivation, fatigue, and a decreased sense of well-being that is identified by sufficient plasma estrogen and low circulating bioavailability of testosterone as well as low sexual desire (libido). Other symptoms include bone loss, decreased muscle strength, and changes in cognition or memory. Bone density may also be affected.

The North American Menopause Society published a comprehensive position statement in September 2005 in its review of testosterone use, which included monitoring, safety, and replacement guidelines and dosages for postmenopausal women. Unfortunately, the U.S. Food and Drug Administration (FDA) has not approved an androgen product for women. It is interesting to note that in Europe a testosterone patch has been approved for use in women.

High levels of testosterone products can have several potential serious side effects including, but not limited to, increased facial and body hair growth (hirsuitism), weight gain, abnormal enlargement of the clitoris (clitoromegaly), hair loss (alopecia), changes in lipid profiles, and liver or hematological changes. Some have reported emotional changes; the safety of androgen in the cancer population has not been adequately studied.

Some of the testosterones successfully used in an off-label setting in some selected women include oral methyltestosteone, transdermal testosterone, topical testosterone prioprionate cream 2%, testosterone gel, and oral dehydroepiandrosterone (DHEA). There are also medications that combine estrogen and androgen. A woman who is taking testosterone off label in an effort to have increased desire or for libido issues should be under the care of a sexual medicine specialist and should have her blood laboratory values monitored closely.

78. Are there other medications that have been used in women for the treatment of sexual complaints?

There are many medications that sexual medicine specialists have used to try to lessen the distress of sexual complaints. It is important to know that none are FDA approved, and there are minimal good scientific data that demonstrate efficacy. However, some of the latest medications include:

- *Phosphodiesterase inhibitors* (Sildenafil, Vardenafil, and Tadalafil) have been approved for the treatment of erectile dysfunction in men. Numerous attempts have been made to show an efficacy in women, but most studies have failed to show any significant benefit in randomized clinical trials. Some potential side effects include headache, uterine contractions, dizziness, hypotension, myocardial infarction (heart attack), stroke, and sudden death. Exciting emerging data may support their use in women who suffer from sexual complaints as a result of hypertension, diabetes, neural and vascular disease, or selective serotonin reuptake inhibitor (SSRI) use.

- *Alprostadil* is a prostaglandin E_1, topical medication that can be applied to the pelvic genital area twice a day to relax arterial smooth blood vessels, causing vasodilatation and increased sensitivity and sexual arousal. Possible side effects include pain to the genitals, lowered blood pressure, and possible temporary fainting (syncope).

- *Bupropion* is a non-SSRI antidepressant, dopamine agonist antidepressant medication with the least sexual side effects. Precautions include insomnia, nervousness, and mild-to-moderate increases in blood pressure as well as a risk of lowering seizure threshold.

Three other medications still under investigation include:

- *Flibanserin*, a 5-HT1A agonist/5-HT2 antagonist. Some of the side effects include nausea, dizziness, fatigue, sleeplessness, and increased bleeding if on a nonsteroidal antiinflammatory drug or aspirin. It is promising for the treatment of female sexual desire disorder.

- *Tibolone* is not available in the United States. It has been shown to reduce hot flashes, increase bone mineral density, and decrease vaginal dryness. The drug does improve desire, but not sexual function. There are some medical concerns regarding the lipid metabolism, hemostasis, and long-term cardiovascular and cancer risks.

- *Bremelanotide* is a melanocortin receptor agonist in phase 2A pilot clinical studies that looked at this medication in premenopausal women diagnosed with female sexual dysfunction and has encouraging results.

Before considering any of these medications, it is crucial to discuss their potential benefits and risks with your oncologist or clinician.

79. What nonhormonal and nonmedication regimes can I use to help with my sexual function?

Because hormones pose serious risks and other medications have some side effects, women may opt to use other types of treatment to help their sexual function. Some helpful sexual products include vaginal moisturizers and lubricants.

The liberal use of local nonmedicated, nonhormonal vaginal moisturizers can provide relief for the symptoms of vaginal atrophy. In addition, the use of water-based vaginal lubricants with intercourse also can relieve vaginal dryness and atrophy. However, some vaginal lubricants contain microbicides, perfumes, coloration, and flavors, and these additives may irritate the

Some vaginal lubricants contain microbicides, perfumes, coloration, and flavors, and these additives may irritate the sensitive atrophic vaginal mucosa.

sensitive atrophic vaginal mucosa. Finally, lubricants may be water or silicone based. Be certain to use a lot of lubricant when attempting intercourse if you are in the middle of treatment for vaginal atrophy or dryness.

80. What is a vaginal dilator?

For women who have had cervical cancer and may suffer from vaginal shortening, vaginal narrowing, and have scar tissue that interferes or prevents penetration and causes vaginal pain, dilators may be helpful. Vaginal dilators may be prescribed as part of your sexual rehabilitation regime. These dilators are graded-size vaginal inserts usually made of plastic or silicone and are often used to facilitate lengthening and widening of the vagina. Dilators can be used on a regular basis and with water- or hormone-based lubricants. Suggested schedules range from once daily for 10 to 15 minutes or at least three times weekly.

Using the vaginal dilator can help expand the vagina and help stretch radiation changes of tissue fibrosis (such as hardening of the vaginal wall tissue) that may have been caused from cancer therapy. Prepare yourself and your environment for dilator therapy. Make certain you will have privacy; many clinicians advise women to use their dilators in the morning hours just before starting the day for several reasons. The dilator should be inserted into the vagina with a generous amount of water-based lubricant. You should lie on your back, bend your knees, and spread your knees apart. With gentle pressure, the vaginal dilator should be inserted into the vagina as deeply as possible while still maintaining some comfort. You should leave the dilator in place for 10 to 15 minutes while remaining on your back. It is often helpful to be distracted by other activities while the dilator is in place, like reading a book, listen to soothing music, or watching a television program. After removing the dilator, it is important to wash it with warm soap and water, dry it with a clean towel, and store it in a safe secure place.

Darlene's comment:

My radiologist gave me my vaginal dilator after I had radiation with a vaginal implant. The dilator is a hard plastic cylinder that is inserted into the vagina for about 10 minutes at a time and is used to help lengthen and widen the vagina.

81. Are there any other aids available to help improve sexual pleasure?

Yes, the Eros Clitoral Stimulator is a sexual device that may be prescribed for patients who have had cervical cancer and other pelvic cancers, such as rectal and vaginal cancers. It is battery operated and has a vacuum suction that attaches to the clitoral area. It is thought to improve **vasocongestion** in the clitoral tissue. Preliminary data show promising results that this device may be helpful in combating arousal difficulties after cervical cancer therapy. It is costly and is available by prescription. Insurance plans vary as to if they will cover the expense.

Vasocongestion
The state in which blood vessels are engorged.

Vibrators can be helpful for women who may need extra vibratory stimulation in the sensitive erotic areas of the vagina and clitoris. Vibrators have proven useful during self-stimulatory behavior and can also be used during sexual foreplay. They are available at local pharmacies, the Internet, and at local sexual paraphernalia shops. Self-stimulators can be used with water-based lubricants. It is important to keep them clean and wash them with warm soap using a sponge or cloth and water before rinsing well. Storage should be in a clean place. Vibrators can be used alone as part of self-erotic exploration, sexual play, or as part of your sexual repertoire. If you share your sexual toys, then it is important to cleanse them in between person use. One Web site (http://drugstore.com) offers home delivery of sexual accessories in a discrete manner, and you will not receive any unwanted e-mails or mailings.

82. Can alternative and complementary medicine improve my sex life?

Women have tried many nonconventional sexual enhancers and therapeutics to facilitate treatment for sexual function complaints and arousal disorders.

Women have tried many nonconventional sexual enhancers and therapeutics to facilitate treatment for sexual function complaints and arousal disorders. There are limited scientifically proven databases containing results of randomized control trial studies that demonstrate beneficial use of these substances for alleviating sexual dysfunction. In fact, many have some concerning side effects. It is best to consult with your physician as to whether a particular product is right for you. This list highlights a few of the more frequently used products.

> *DHEA.* Some studies show that a low level (50 mg/day) of DHEA can improve the frequency of sexual thoughts, sexual interest, and sexual satisfaction over a placebo. It can be prescribed at a starting dosage of 50 mg/day and has shown to increase libido in some women. Caution should be used with this because it can increase androgens, decrease high-density lipoprotein, (HDL), decrease sex-hormone

binding globulin (SHBG), and high levels of DHEA are correlated with increased risk of cardiovascular disease. Caution should be used because these products are not monitored by the FDA and label claims may not accurately reflect the actual DHEA content in the product.

Avlimil is an herbal 756-milligram per day supplemental tablet consisting of sage leaf, red raspberry leaf, capsicum pepper, licorice root, bayberry fruit, damiana leaf, valeriana root, ginger root, black cohosh root, isoflavones, kudzu root extract, and red clover extract (see www.avlimil.com for the comprehensive details). The product package insert states that it is a nonsynthetic, nonhormonal supplement that does not contain estrogen, progesterone, testosterone, or steroid hormones. However, the fine print of the labeling states: "If estrogen levels are low, Isoflavones are reported to act as 'weak estrogens'." Avlimil is presumed to increase sexual satisfaction by increasing genital pelvic blood flow and by promoting relaxation.

Arginmax is a daily supplement that claims to enhance a women's sexual response by promoting genital pelvic blood flow and promoting relaxation. It is a blend of L-arginine, Korean ginseng, ginkgo biloba, damiana, calcium, iron, and 14 vitamins. The product claims to increase smooth muscular relaxation, promote vascular dilatation, and enhance clitoral engorgement and vaginal lubrication.

83. Can changing my diet improve sexual function?

Although patients try many different foods, such as chocolate, ginseng, oysters, and popular sexual-enhancing diets to facilitate improved sexual function, none have been shown in randomized clinical trials to be beneficial for correcting female sexual complaints.

PART TWELVE

Fertility After Cervical Cancer

Have there been successful pregnancies after women underwent a radical trachelectomy?

What can be done to preserve my ability to have children in the future?

Can I adopt children after a diagnosis of cancer?

More . . .

84. Have there been successful pregnancies after women underwent a radical trachelectomy?

Yes. In one report, there were 50 pregnancies among 72 women treated with radical trachelectomy for stage IA or IB disease. However, while it is possible to carry a pregnancy after a trachelectomy, the risks of bleeding, spontaneous abortion or miscarriage, or prematurity are real with a quoted rate of first trimester miscarriage at 16 percent and of second trimester miscarriage at 4 percent. Still, 72 percent of pregnancies reach the third trimester and 8 percent go past 32 weeks. The vast majority of children born to mothers who have had a radical trachelectomy are reported to be developing normally.

85. What can be done to preserve my ability to have children in the future?

If you are not a candidate for a radical trachelectomy, you may be a candidate for a procedure called **ovarian transposition**. In this surgery, the ovaries are surgically moved away from the radiation area, which can minimize their radiation exposure. The success in maintaining function in the ovaries can range from 60 to 100 percent, although pregnancy rates are lower.

Ovarian transposition

Moving the ovaries to another location. Usually, it is done in women who require radiation as a way to spare the ovaries from the toxic effects of radiation and hopefully to preserve fertility.

Darlene's comment:

You may choose to harvest eggs and then have the embryo inserted into a surrogate. I tried to harvest eggs, but none would mature. My doctor took a piece of my ovary and froze it; however, I'm not sure if there is anything that we could do with it. I think the statistics for achieving pregnancy are very low.

86. Can I adopt children after a diagnosis of cancer?

Most adoption agencies do not rule out cancer survivors as parents but do require full disclosure of your medical history and recent medical examinations.

Most adoption agencies do not rule out cancer survivors as parents but do require full disclosure of your medical history and recent medical examinations. Others may require your oncologist to write a letter of support and a declaration that you are cancer free; still others may require you to be cancer free for 5 years before considering you as a potential parent. It is important that you work with specialists in the adoption arena who have a good record of working with cancer survivors. Adoption can also take a significant amount of time and effort, leading to psychological and emotional stress. Recognizing that the pathway to adoption can be a long and winding road is important, as is finding a strong support system including your friends, family, and adoption specialists.

Surrogacy

A type of parenting agreement in which one woman carries a pregnancy for someone else.

Traditional surrogacy

A parenting agreement in which the embryo that is carried by a surrogate came from the surrogate's own egg.

Gestational surrogacy

A parenthood option in which a woman (the surrogate) carries a pregnancy for another person. In this arrangement, the egg is from a donor, not from the surrogate.

87. What are other options for parenting?

Beyond carrying your own biological child, other alternatives for parenthood are more commonly being utilized. Some of these include using the eggs of volunteer women, which can be fertilized through in-vitro fertilization for transfer into yourself. If you cannot carry a pregnancy due to surgery or other treatment for cervical cancer, another option is to ask another woman to carry your baby in a **surrogacy**. In a **traditional surrogacy** agreement, the woman donating her eggs also carries the child. In a **gestational surrogacy** agreement, the egg donor and the woman carrying the pregnancy are different women. Egg donors can be known or anonymous and are frequently young women. They must be screened psychologically and medically to ensure they understand what egg donation entails and to ensure that they are healthy and free of sexually transmitted diseases. Women looking into becoming a surrogate also undergo both mental health and medical screening to ensure they are psychologically and physically prepared to carry a pregnancy. In addition, surrogacy laws vary by state, so using an attorney to assist in legal arrangements is important.

Darlene's comment:

Adoption is a great option. There is always going to be a child who needs a mother. My husband and I know that adoption is a choice that we can both agree on. I have friends who have an adopted as well as a biological child. They say that they love each child equally. There is no difference in the care and the love that you will have for an adopted child. Foster parenting may also be an option if one cannot financially afford to adopt.

PART THIRTEEN

Prevention and Screening

Are there guidelines on when and how often Pap tests should be done?

Are there special guidelines for older women?

Are women who are HIV infected followed differently?

More . . .

88. Are there guidelines on when and how often Pap tests should be done?

Pap tests are among the most successful screening tests in the world, and in the United States have led to a decrease in the number of new cases of cancer diagnosed in the country each year. The American Cancer Society recommends that Pap tests begin about 3 years after the onset of sexual activity, but no later than the age of 21. If three consecutive Pap tests are negative, a woman can consider being screened less frequently; for example, every 2–3 years instead of annually.

The American Cancer Society recommends that Pap tests begin about 3 years after the onset of sexual activity, but no later than the age of 21.

Following treatment for cervical cancer, women are closely followed for recurrence. The National Comprehensive Cancer Network recommends surveillance using Pap tests and physical exams every 3 months for the first year, every 4 months in the second year, then every 6 months to year 5. Beyond that, Pap tests should be performed annually. Other considerations for cancer surveillance include bloodwork every 6 months and a chest X-ray annually, but these are not strict recommendations and should be discussed with your doctor.

89. Are there special guidelines for older women?

Women over 70 who have had three negative Pap tests in a row and no history of abnormal Pap tests in the prior 10 years may not need continued screening and can discuss stopping screening with their doctors. This is simply because cervical cancer is rare among older women who have been screened, and the quality of the samples that are taken as a woman ages decreases due to the physical changes in the vagina and the cervix.

PREVENTION AND SCREENING

90. Are women who are HIV infected followed differently?

Women infected with HIV should undergo a Pap test twice the first year after they are diagnosed, and then annually. Other women who are immunocompromised or are at an increased risk for cervical cancer because their mother took a drug called diethylstilbestrol while pregnant with them should be screened annually as well, even if prior Pap tests are normal.

91. If I had my uterus removed, do I still need to have Pap tests?

Fibroids

Noncancerous tumors of the uterus.

If you had your uterus removed (called a hysterectomy) for noncancer-related reasons, such as for **fibroids** (noncancer muscle outgrowths from the uterus) or due to excessive bleeding, then there is no reason to have the Pap tests performed. However, if you had a hysterectomy due to cancer of the cervix, vagina, vulva, ovaries, or uterus, then you should continue to be screened as noted in Question 94.

92. How do vaccines work?

Vaccines work by teaching the immune system to recognize and attack bacteria or viruses that can cause disease in the human body. Many types of vaccines are administered today, most of which are administered beginning shortly after birth and continuing through young adulthood.

The method of training the body to recognize disease-causing bacteria or viruses is by exposing the immune system to either a portion of the bacteria or virus, or the whole bacteria or virus that has been made unable to cause disease. A classic example of a vaccine that is made from an inactive virus is the polio vaccine. An example of a vaccine that is made from a replica of a portion of a virus is the hepatitis B vaccine. The hepatitis B vaccine is made by implanting that part of the hepatitis B virus DNA that causes growth of the hepatitis B virus shell into an animal cell. The animal cell then produces many copies of the shell of the virus without the active particle inside. Once it is injected, this shell is recognized by the immune system without the risk of contracting the actual disease and as such, the vaccine causes an immune response. Immune cells in the body learn to recognize the vaccine so that when a person is exposed to the real disease-causing bacteria or virus, the memory of how to respond is already prepared and the disease can be avoided.

93. What is the cervical cancer vaccine?

The cervical cancer vaccine is a vaccine developed to protect against certain types of human papillomavirus (HPV). HPV is found in 100 percent of cervical cancers. HPV can also be found in high rates in penile, vaginal, vulvar, head and neck, throat, and anal cancers. Along with cancer, HPV is associated with genital warts and other precancerous lesions of the cervix, vagina, and vulva.

HPV can also be found in high rates in penile, vaginal, vulvar, head and neck, throat, and anal cancers.

There are approximately 100 different strains, or types, of HPV. Some have a higher risk for causing cancer, while others have a higher risk for causing genital warts or precancerous change. HPV types 16 and 18 have the greatest association with cervical cancers, accounting for 75 percent of all new cervical cancer cases. These types also are associated with a high risk of severe precancerous changes. HPV types 6 and 11 are frequently associated with genital warts and other lower grade pre-cancerous changes.

The HPV vaccine currently approved is Gardasil. It is an inactive vaccine, and there is no risk of becoming infected with HPV by receiving the vaccine. The currently approved HPV vaccine is designed to prevent the effects of HPV types 6, 11, 16, and 18 on the cervix, vagina, and vulva of women. Encouraging results suggest that cross-protection occurs to other HPV strains. Based on studies already performed, the HPV vaccine will prevent approximately 75 percent of cervical cancer overall and practically 100 percent of cervical cancer, genital warts, and precancerous changes of the cervix, vagina, and vulva caused by the four HPV types just mentioned.

Another vaccine in late development is Cervarix, which was filed for approval by the FDA and may be approved in the very near future. It is designed against HPV 16 and 18. Like Gardasil, it also has been reported to offer cross-protection. **Table 3** compares both of these vaccines.

94. Will the vaccine mean I don't need to get Pap tests anymore?

The HPV vaccine is designed to prevent infection by HPV types 6, 11, 16, and 18. Unfortunately, there are many other HPV types that can infect the cervix, vagina, and vulva. These other HPV types can cause cervical cancer as well as genital warts and other pre-cancerous changes on the cervix, vagina, or vulva. For that reason, Pap tests are still recommended as a method of screening for these diseases.

Table 3 HPV Vaccines: Gardasil versus Cervarix

	Gardasil	Cervarix
Manufacturer	Merck	GlasoSmithKline
Type	Tetravalent	Bivalent
HPV-strain VLPs*	6, 11, 16, 18	16, 18
Adjuvant used	Aluminum phosphate	ASO4 (aluminum salt plus monophosphoryl lipid A)
Production	Saccharomyces cerevesiae (yeast)	Recombinant baculovirus–infected cells
FDA status	Approved as pro-phylaxis against cervical cancer and against cutaneous genital warts	Filed for United States approval, March 2007
Vaccination schedule	3 injections at 0, 2, and 6 months	3 injections at 0, 1, and 6 months
Efficacy:		
• protection against infection	100%	90%
• protection against CIN2+ lesions	98%	
Cross Protection	31, 33, 35, 39, 45, 51, 52, 56, 58, 59	31, 33, 35, 39, 45, 51, 52, 56, 58, 59, 66, 68

*VLP: virus-like particle

95. If I have been infected with HPV, will the vaccine protect me from getting cervical cancer?

The vaccine is designed to be effective only against HPV types 6, 11, 16, and 18. Some women infected with HPV may have one or more of these types. For example, if a woman has HPV type 18, the vaccine will not protect her against the effects of type 18. However, it will provide her protection against the other three types. The initial studies with these vaccines included some patients who had an infection with one or more of these HPV types. There was a definite benefit proven for these patients. Based on the evidence, the vaccine is recommended in women with a prior or current HPV infection.

96. How old should you be to be vaccinated?

The American Cancer Society has put out recommendations for who should be vaccinated and how old you should be (**Table 4**). Vaccine is currently approved for use in females from ages 9 to 26. Use of the vaccine for women older than 26 would be an off-label use of the vaccine and would be an individualized decision between the patient and her healthcare provider.

Table 4 American Cancer Society Recommendations for HPV Vaccination

- Routine HPV vaccination is recommended for females aged 11 to 12 years.
- Females as young as age 9 years may receive HPV vaccination.
- HPV vaccination is also recommended for females aged 13 to 18 years.
- A decision about whether a woman aged 19 to 26 years should receive the vaccine should be based on an informed discussion with the woman and her healthcare provider.
- HPV vaccination is not recommended for women over age 26 or males.
- Cervical cytology screening should continue in vaccinated and unvaccinated women.

Source: Adapted from Saslow D, Castle PE, Cox TJ, et al. American Cancer Society Guideline for Human Papillomavirus (HPV) Vaccine Use to Prevent Cervical Cancer and Its Precursors. *CA Cancer J Clin.* 2007;57:7–28.

97. What are the side effects of the vaccine?

The most common side effects of the vaccine are redness, swelling, and pain at the injection site, similar to most vaccinations. A small fraction of women may experience a fever and flu-like symptoms. There have been a few reports of patients being allergic to the vaccine. In the long-term follow-up of patients on the original trials, there have been no long-term side effects.

The vaccine is contraindicated in pregnancy but not in lactating women. If a woman receives the vaccine and then discovers she is pregnant, she should report it to her healthcare provider as soon as possible. The healthcare provider should report it to the manufacturer. A registry of pregnant patients who have received the vaccine is being compiled to assess for any effects on the developing fetus. To date, there have been no associated birth defects.

98. How long are you protected after you've had the vaccine?

The vaccine is designed to offer lifetime protection from HPV. The question as to whether a booster injection will be required remains yet to be answered. With greater than 5 years of follow-up of the patients originally vaccinated on the trial, there has been no need for a booster demonstrated.

The vaccine is a three-injection series administered over a 6-month span. Although it is possible that some women will gain immunity after only one or two injections, it is unsafe to assume that a woman will be protected until after she has completed the three-shot series.

99. Why would I get a vaccine if Pap tests are so effective?

Pap tests are a form of secondary cancer prevention. They do not address the fundamental causes of cervical cancer, most common of which is HPV. To prevent the cause of cervical cancer from infecting a patient, or primary prevention, is the purpose of the HPV vaccine.

Approximately 20 percent of women with cervical cancer will have had a recent false negative Pap test.

Unfortunately, Pap tests are not perfect. Approximately 20 percent of women with cervical cancer will have had a recent false negative Pap test. This is by no means the fault of the healthcare provider obtaining the sample or the one interpreting the results. There is just an inherent lack of accuracy within the test that is only overcome because the test is repeated on a relatively frequent (annual) basis.

Another major problem with relying on Pap tests is compliance. Failure to have the Pap test done at the recommended interval occurs either because the patient did not pursue it or there is a shortage of providers or funding to do the test for patients. Although never meant to replace the need for Pap tests, vaccination will help to prevent a certain number of cancers annually even for noncompliant patients.

100. Where can I get more information?

There are numerous resources available for you or your loved ones regarding cervical cancer. Fortunately, the Internet has put a significant amount of resources within reach for many women. A listing of useful resources regarding cervical cancer is presented here:

About Cervical Neoplasia, Prevention, and Workup:

American Society for Colposcopy and Cervical Pathology:
www.asccp.org

American College of Obstetrics and Gynecology:
www.acog.org

About HPV:

Centers for Disease Control and Prevention: www.cdc.gov/

National Women's Health Information Center:
www.4woman.gov/

About Cervical Cancer:

National Cancer Institute:
www.cancer.gov/cancertopics/types/cervical/

American Cancer Society: www.cancer.org/

American Society of Clinical Oncology: www.asco.org

National Cervical Cancer Coalition: www.nccc-online.org

Gynecologic Cancer Foundation: www.thegcf.org

Society of Gynecologic Oncologists: www.sgo.org

Treatment Options:

Clinical trials: www.clinical-trials.gov

Gynecologic Oncology Group: www.gog.org

Survivorship:

National Coalition for Cancer Survivorship:
www.canceradvocacy.org

Lance Armstrong Foundation: www.livestrong.org

NCI Office of Cancer Survivorship: dccps.nci.gov/ocs/

Sexual Health:

The Women's Sexual Health Foundation: www.twshf.org

The International Society for the Study of Women's Sexual
Health: www.isswsh.org

North American Menopause Society: www.menopause.org

PREVENTION AND SCREENING

Fertility:

FertileHope: www.fertilehope.org

Darlene's comment:

The American Cancer Society, my physician, and the library are all places where I looked for the information I needed.

A

Ablation: Removing tissue by surgery or any other means.

Acupuncture: A traditional Chinese practice of treating a health condition or medical state by inserting needles into the skin at specific points to unblock the flow of energy.

Adenocarcinoma: A glandular-type of cancer that arises from different parts of the body, including the cervix.

Apoptosis: The process of programmed cell death.

Aromatherapy: An integrative care practice that uses oils from plants to treat physical or psychological conditions. These oils are either inhaled or used in massage.

B

Best supportive care: A treatment principle concentrated on the relief of symptoms from a disease, as opposed to treating the disease itself.

Bioidentical hormones: Hormonal preparations, usually animal or plant derived, that have a similar chemical structure to a human's naturally occurring hormones.

Biologic modifiers: Drugs or compounds that aim to stimulate or to restore the ability of the immune system to fight disease or infections.

Biphosphonate: A class of drugs that are used to prevent or treat osteoporosis or bone degeneration.

Brachytherapy: The technique of giving radiation by placing the radioactive source directly inside or next to the area of treatment. In cervical cancer, the source generally is placed inside the vagina so that the cervix can be treated specifically.

C

Cancer: A disease characterized by uncontrolled cell growth that ultimately causes destruction of normal healthy tissue.

Cardinal ligament: A fibrous band attached to the cervix and the vagina laterally, extending to the uterus, to provide support. It also contains the blood vessels to the pelvis.

Cerclage: A stitch placed into and around the cervix of a pregnant woman to help reduce the possibility of miscarriage.

Cervical canal: Also known as the endocervical canal, it is the tunnel that connects the uterus to the vagina.

Cervical intraepithelial neoplasia (CIN): Abnormal cell growth within the cervix. It can range from low-risk changes (CIN-1) to more abnormal changes (CIN-2 and CIN-3). These are also referred to as squamous intraepithelial lesions. Although not cancer, these changes can progress into cancer.

Cervix: From the Latin for neck, it is the lowermost part of the uterus that protrudes into the vagina.

Chemical menopause: Induction of menopause by the use of treatments that are toxic to the ovaries; includes such treatments as radiation, chemotherapy, or hormonal.

Chemotherapy: Medications that cause cells to stop dividing; used in the treatment of cancer.

Clitoris: A woman's highly sensitive pelvic organ that is associated with orgasm.

Cold knife cone biopsy: Also known as a cone biopsy, this technique enables sampling of abnormal cervical tissue that is seen during examination by the use of a scalpel. A cone-shaped portion of the cervix is removed.

Colonoscopy: A diagnostic test for evaluating the colon.

Colostomy: A surgical procedure in which a part of the colon is connected to the anterior abdominal wall. The opening of the colostomy at the wall is termed a stoma and is the means by which stool is passed.

Colposcopy: A diagnostic procedure performed by gynecologists to look at the cervix more closely. It is performed with a colposcope, which is a large electric microscope that helps the doctor see the cervix more clearly.

Cone biopsy: *See* cold knife cone biopsy.

Cryotherapy: The treatment of abnormal tissue by freezing.

CT scans: Computed tomography scans used as a diagnostic imaging test.

D

Differentiation: The biologic process by which a cell becomes a specific type.

DNA: Deoxyribonucleic acid, the building blocks of cells.

DNR order: A "Do Not Resuscitate" order, which communicates a person's wishes not to be revived or kept alive through artificial means.

Dosage: The amount or volume to be taken, as generally prescribed by a healthcare provider.

Dyspareunia: Pain with sexual intercourse.

Dysplasia: Abnormal changes in cells.

E

Endocervical canal: *See* cervical canal.

Endocervical curettage (ECC): A sampling of the internal cervix obtained during a colposcopy. The sampling is taken by scraping the inner portion of the cervix, which cannot be seen during a pelvic exam.

Endometrial biopsy: The process of obtaining tissue from the uterine lining.

Epithelial cell abnormality: A result that may be reported on a Pap test that signifies a change is present in cells that might require further evaluation by the doctor.

Estrogen: A steroid hormone produced mainly in the ovaries; it is the primary female sex hormone.

Excision: Removal of an area of concern (whether it be an area of tumor growth or of abnormal growth) usually done with surgery.

External os: The opening that connects the uterus and cervix to the vagina.

F

Fecal occult blood test: A noninvasive test that checks for blood in the stool.

Female androgen insufficiency syndrome: A constellation of symptoms attributed to low testosterone levels in women including unexplained fatigue, decreased well-being, lack of energy or motivation, and decreased sexual function.

Fibroids: Noncancerous tumors of the uterus.

G

Gestational surrogacy: A parenthood option in which a woman (the surrogate) carries a pregnancy for another person. In this arrangement, the egg is from a donor, not from the surrogate.

Glandular: Of or pertaining to a gland.

H

Healthcare proxy: Also known as a durable power of attorney for healthcare, it is a legally named person who is tasked with making medical decisions for a person if that person is unable to make them.

Hematogenous dissemination: The process by which cancer spreads through the bloodstream to other parts of the body.

Hematogenous spread: *See* hematogenous dissemination.

Hormone therapy (HT): The use of medications to modify or replace the hormones a body makes or lacks. In the case of cancer, hormone therapy may be those medications that block hormones from feeding a cancer cell. However, in the case of hot flashes, it may denote medications given to enhance low levels of hormones that result from menopause.

Hospice: A philosophy for care at the end of life, aiming to provide patients with comfort, dignity, and quality in the last phases of an illness.

Human papillomavirus (HPV): The virus associated with genital tract infections, including most cases of cervical dysplasia and cancer.

Hysterectomy: The surgical removal of the uterus.

I

Internal os: The internal narrowing of the uterine cavity that serves as a passageway from the external os into the uterus.

L

Laser: A technique in which light is the source for vaporizing and removing abnormal tissue.

Libido: A person's sex drive.

Living will: A legal document that specifies a person's advance wishes in case the person is not able to consent to (or refuse) treatment. It is also known as an advance directive.

Loop electrosurgical excision procedure (LEEP): A surgical technique in which an electrically charged loop of wire is passed across the surface of the cervix, resulting in the removal of abnormal tissue.

Luteinizing hormone (LH): A hormone produced by the pituitary gland that is necessary for reproductive function. Rises in LH trigger an egg to be released from the ovary.

Lymph nodes: A part of the lymphatic system, these are glands composed of lymphocytes that act as the filtration system of the body.

Lymphatic spread: The use of the body's filtration system by cancer cells to spread.

Lymphatic system: A network of channels, nodes, and vessels that function as a transport system of lymph fluid. It functions as a major component of the immune system.

Lymphedema: The backup of lymph fluid due to an obstruction or the removal of lymph nodes that results in the swelling of the affected body part.

Lymphocele: A sac of lymph fluid usually as the result of surgery and/or damage to the lymphatic system.

M

Mammography: A special X-ray of the breast that is used as a screening tool for breast cancer.

Meditation: A complementary medicine practice of concentrated attention toward a single point of reference.

Menopause: The permanent end of a woman's menstrual cycle.

Metastatic: Cancer that has spread beyond the place where it started.

Microinvasive: In cervical cancer, it refers to the microscopic finding of cancer cells that have penetrated the usual border in small collections. It represents the earliest evidence of invasion.

Music therapy: A complementary therapy practice using music to help psychologic or emotional adjustment before, during, or after cancer is diagnosed.

Mutations: Cellular changes that can predispose to developing cancer.

N

Neoadjuvant chemotherapy: The use of cancer drugs as first treatment aimed at reducing the size or involvement of cancer.

O

Osteonecrosis: The process describing bone death.

Osteoporosis: Bony degeneration; also known as osteoarthritis.

Ovarian transposition: Moving the ovaries to another location. Usually, it is done in women who require radiation as a way to spare the ovaries from the toxic effects of radiation and hopefully to preserve fertility.

P

Palliation: To provide comfort.

Palliative care: A healthcare model for which attention to symptoms is as important as (or may even replace) the treatment of the disease itself.

Papanicolaou (Pap) test: A cervical test that is used to screen for cervical changes or cancer.

Para-aortic area: The region near the aorta; it generally refers to a group of nodes that can be involved by cancer of the cervix.

Parametria: The connective tissue and fat that lies adjacent to the uterus.

Pelvic exenteration: A radical surgical procedure that involves removal of the pelvic organs, which may include the bladder (anterior exenteration) and/or the rectum and anus (posterior exenteration). It is performed as a curative procedure in women with recurrent cervical cancer.

Pelvic lymph nodes: A group of nodes that lie within the pelvis. These are at high risk of being involved with cervical cancer.

Perimenopausal: The time in which women are having irregular periods, right before the periods completely stop.

Placebo: In clinical trials, it refers to the use of pills that possess no medicinal properties.

Positron emission test (PET) scan: A radiologic test that uses information on the metabolism of cells to differentiate normal from abnormal tissue. Highly active tissue on a PET scan in a patient with cervical cancer can indicate that cancer has spread to that area.

Proctoscopy: A technique using a scope to examine the rectum, anus, and colon.

Progesterone: A hormone in women that is required for normal periods, maintaining pregnancy, and the development of the fetus.

Pyelogram: A radiologic test that specifically looks at the kidney and ureters.

R

Radical trachelectomy: A surgical procedure for early cervical cancer that involves removing the cervix only. It is a technique that allows women to maintain the potential of carrying a pregnancy.

Recurrence: Cancer that has returned despite treatment.

Reflexology: A complementary medicine practice that uses massage, squeezing, or pushing (normally of the feet or hands) to encourage positive effects on other body parts or provide a general sense of well-being.

Reiki: A spiritual practice that uses healing energy to improve symptoms or treat conditions.

Remission: A designation of being cancer free.

Roots: The finding that cancer has involved deeper into normal tissue or extended outside the place it started.

S

Sentinel lymph node biopsy: A technique using dye and/or a radioactive substance injected into the tumor with the aim of identifying its drainage pattern in the lymph system. The first node(s) that are identified are termed the sentinel node.

149

Speculum: A medical examination tool that enables a doctor to view the cervix.

Squamous: A type of cell that lines the skin and external body surfaces.

Surgical menopause: The complete stop of a woman's periods that occurs as a result of the removal of the ovaries.

Surrogacy: A type of parenting agreement in which one woman carries a pregnancy for someone else.

Survivorship medicine: The medical practice aimed at addressing the physical needs, long-term health, and life changes that result following the diagnosis and treatment for cancer.

T

Tandem: In radiation, it is the tube that is inserted into the vagina to allow direct radiation of the cervix.

Testosterone: A sexual hormone produced in the ovaries that is important in normal sexual functioning.

Traditional surrogacy: A parenting agreement in which the embryo that is carried by a surrogate came from the surrogate's own egg.

Transformation zone: The area in the cervix marked by the transition between the outside of the cervix (lined by squamous cells) and the cervical canal (lined by columnar cells). It is also known as the squamo-columnar junction.

Transvaginal ultrasound: A radiology test in which the probe (on the ultrasound) is inserted directly into the vagina. It is the most accurate way to evaluate a woman's reproductive organs.

Tumor: A cancerous mass.

Twilight: A state induced with medication that allows sedation, making invasive procedures more comfortable. Ideally, medications will induce a state of sleep in which the person closes the eyes and rests while the procedure is performed.

U

Ureters: Tubes that connect the kidneys to the bladder for passing urine.

Urostomy: An artificial opening that allows urine to pass. It is created surgically if a person needs to have the bladder removed during an exenteration.

Uterus: The female reproductive organ in which pregnancy occurs.

V

Vagina: That part of the female genital tract that connects the uterus to the external vulva.

Vaginal cuff: The part created by a surgeon at the top of the vagina following removal of the cervix.

Vaginal dilators: Medical plastic applicators that help restore the vaginal muscles so that they are more adaptable.

Vaginal fibrosis: The narrowing or scarring of the vagina. It can make sex extremely painful for women.

Vaginal vault: The area at the top of the vagina, adjacent to the cervix.

Vaginismus: An involuntary tightening of the vaginal muscles when the vagina is penetrated. This action can cause significant pain.

Vasocongestion: The state in which blood vessels are engorged.

Villoglandular carcinoma: A specific type of invasive cancer that typically does not spread to the surrounding tissues of the cervix. It is a less aggressive variant of cervical cancer.

Vulva: The external female genitals that are seen when a woman is naked.

Y

Yoga: The spiritual practice aiming to unite the consciousness with universal consciousness to achieve harmony.